Journal of
Health Politics,
Policy

T0257064

Editor Jonathan Oberlander, University of North Carolina at Chapel Hill
Associate Editors Nicholas Bagley, University of Michigan; Sarah E.
Gollust, University of Minnesota; Helen Levy, University of Michigan;
Elizabeth Rigby, George Washington University
Book Review Editor Miriam J. Laugesen, Columbia University
Special Section Editors Beneath the Surface: Joseph White, Case
Western Reserve University; Tracking Health Reform: Heather Howard,
Princeton University, and Frank J. Thompson, Rutgers University
Social Media Editor Harold A. Pollack, University of Chicago
Managing Editor Jed P. Cohen
Former Editors Ralph A. Straetz, New York University; Theodore
R. Marmor, Yale University; Lawrence D. Brown, Columbia University;
James A. Morone, Brown University; Mark A. Peterson, University
of California, Los Angeles; Mark Schlesinger, Yale University;
Michael S. Sparer, Columbia University; Colleen M. Grogan,
University of Chicago; Eric M. Patashnik, Brown University

Volume 45, Number 2, April 2020
Published by Duke University Press

Board of Editors

Elizabeth M. Armstrong, Princeton University
Daniel Béland, McGill University
David Blumenthal, Harvard University
Andrea Louise Campbell, Massachusetts Institute of Technology
Daniel Carpenter, Harvard University
Norman Daniels, Harvard University
Judith Feder, Georgetown University
Daniel M. Fox, Milbank Memorial Fund
David M. Frankford, Rutgers University
Erika Franklin-Fowler, Wesleyan University
Marie Gottschalk, University of Pennsylvania
Scott L. Greer, University of Michigan
Michael K. Gusmano, Hastings Center
Mark Hall, Wake Forest University
Richard Hall, University of Michigan
Allison K. Hoffman, University of Pennsylvania
Lawrence R. Jacobs, University of Minnesota
David K. Jones, Boston University
Timothy Stoltzfus Jost, Washington and Lee University
Rogan Kersh, Wake Forest University
Anna Kirkland, University of Michigan
Lars Thorup Larsen, Aarhus University
Julia Lynch, University of Pennsylvania
Hans Maarse, Maastricht University
Wendy Mariner, Boston University
Rick Mayes, University of Richmond
David Mechanic, Rutgers University
Jamila Michener, Cornell University
Edward Miller, University of Massachusetts Boston
Kieke G. H. Okma, New York University
Adam Oliver, London School of Economics and Political Science
Thomas Oliver, University of Wisconsin, Madison
Julianna Pacheco, University of Iowa
Jill Quadagno, Florida State University
Thomas H. Rice, University of California, Los Angeles
Marc Rodwin, Suffolk University
Theda Skocpol, Harvard University
Steven Rathgeb Smith, American Political Science Association
Deborah A. Stone, Brandeis University
Sandra J. Tanenbaum, Ohio State University
Sue Tolleson-Rinehart, University of North Carolina, Chapel Hill
Carolyn Tuohy, University of Toronto

Contents

Special Issue
The Politics of the Opioid Epidemic

Special Issue Editors: Susan L. Moffitt and Eric M. Patashnik

Commentary

Introduction:
The Politics of the Opioid Epidemic

Susan L. Moffitt
Brown University

Opioids' impacts in the United States over the past two decades have been vast, profound, and complex. High death rates, overdose rates, and addiction rates manifested across varied geographies, ages, and racial and ethnic groups (CDC n.d.; Scholl et al. 2019). Opioids impaired economic productivity, strained health care systems, created new demands on the criminal justice system, and burdened family and community networks (NIDA n.d.-a). Varied forms of opioids—prescription drugs, heroin, fentanyl—contributed to the epidemic, emerged from different distribution sources, and presented different implications for various parts of public health systems.

Medical scholarship has made considerable strides in learning about the mechanisms that underlie opioid addiction, the correlates for its incidence, and promising forms of medical interventions (Williams et al. 2013; Walley et al. 2013; Schwartz et al. 2013). Public health scholarship has revealed aspects of medical policy and practice that contributed to the opioid epidemic, including physicians' prescribing practices and weak regulatory oversight from the Food and Drug Administration (Hadlad et al. 2017, 2019; Zettler, Riley, and Kesselheim 2018). Yet, we know much less about the roles that politics and governments at all levels of the system have played in abetting the epidemic. What has US policy and practice done in response to the current predicament, and what are key lessons for policy and practice moving forward? The director of the National Institutes for Health and the director of the National Institute on Drug Abuse have called for "all scientific hands on deck" to effectively address opioid addiction

Journal of Health Politics, Policy and Law, Vol. 45, No. 2, April 2020
DOI 10.1215/03616878-8004838   © 2020 by Duke University Press

and its impact (Volkow and Collins 2017a, 2017b). This special issue of the *Journal of Health Politics, Policy and Law* represents a political science "all hands on deck" approach to understand the complex governmental and political terrain in which the opioid epidemic has unfolded. Underlying medical problems reside in political representation problems, social and economic inequality problems, and bureaucratic adaptation problems. By bringing together scholars from different theoretical perspectives and by examining different levels of government engagement with opioids, this issue considers how addressing questions about opioids also provides new insights on enduring features of US politics and policy, including the power of race, the development of the conservative welfare state, and the challenge of crafting interventions that work on the frontlines.

The politics of race have figured prominently in national responses to opioids. Since death rates associated with opioid use have been higher among whites than other groups (CDC 2018; NIDA n.d.-b), have legislators been more likely to pursue less punitive, more public health–oriented policies in response to opioids in contrast to more punitive criminal justice policies pursued for other drug epidemics? To start this special issue, Jin Woo Kim, Evan Morgan, and Brendan Nyhan compare the opioid era with the crack cocaine era to test whether the policy response to opioids has been less punitive than the response to crack, and whether differences in policy responses are associated with race. Using original data on district-level drug-related deaths and (co)sponsorship of legislation in the House of Representatives on illegal drugs, they find policy makers were more likely to introduce punitive drug-related bills during the crack era and were more likely to introduce treatment-oriented bills in the opioid era. Their results also suggest the relationship between district-level drug deaths and subsequent sponsorship of treatment-oriented legislation is greater for opioid deaths than for cocaine-related deaths and for white victims than for black victims. Their results demonstrate the persistence of racial inequalities and double standards in US drug policy.

The next question this issue addresses is, Does this trend that emerges in Congress of less punitive, more public health approaches for opioids relative to other epidemics also extend to media coverage? Carmel Shachar, Tess Wise, Gali Katznelson, and Andrea Louise Campbell provide additional evidence on racial inequalities through differences in the ways that media have portrayed the opioid and crack epidemics. Drawing on newspapers from across the country and over time, they systematically evaluate how each epidemic was framed in public discourse. They find that articles on the opioid epidemic are more likely to use medical terminology while articles on the crack cocaine epidemic used criminal justice terms more frequently. The differences in how the media have framed the two epidemics reveal additional ways in which race may play a role in public policy responses and outreach.

Racial politics also emerge in public opinion on policy alternatives. By assessing individuals who perceive themselves to be health policy losers, Sarah E. Gollust and Joanne M. Miller depart from and extend conventional scholarship that focuses on perceptions of being a political loser. Gollust and Miller find that whites who perceive themselves to be on the losing side of public health had less empathetic responses to the opioid crisis. Perceiving oneself to be a political loser, however, was unrelated to attitudes about addressing opioids. Their findings suggest how perceptions that one's racial group has lost ground in the public health context could have down-stream political consequences.

How has partisanship played a role in responses to the opioid epidemic, and what do these responses reveal about the development of the conservative welfare state in America? Colleen M. Grogan, Clifford S. Bersamira, Phillip M. Singer, Bikki Tran Smith, Harold A. Pollack, Christina M. Andrews, and Amanda J. Abraham take up these questions and offer new insights on the conservative welfare state. Their analysis of the intersection of state Medicaid policies and opioid assistance reveals that actions in Republican-led state policy do not mirror Republican oppositional rhetoric and proposals at the federal level. Challenging conventional theories of welfare state retrenchment, their findings suggest conservatives rely on program fragmentation to both expand and retrench benefits, not only to retrench programs.

Given the scope and complexity of the opioid epidemic, where do we go from here? Information campaigns constitute a commonly used policy approach to public health problems. Yet, Paul F. Testa, Susan L. Moffitt, and Marie Schenk demonstrate how experimental approaches that assess the impact of information campaigns may misestimate their effects by failing to account for respondents' willingness to receive new information, policy, and research. Using a doubly randomized survey experiment, Testa and his colleagues examine how willingness to seek new information shapes the way members of the public update their preferences about policies related to the opioid epidemic. Among those respondents likely to receive information, treatment has a large positive effect on increasing support for policies to address the opioid epidemic. Among those who would avoid this information, preferences appear to be unmoved by treatment. These effects would be missed by standard experimental designs and highlight the importance of access to and receptiveness toward new information.

Yet, information campaigns constitute only one component of addressing complex policy problems, like the opioid epidemic. Patricia Strach, Katie Zuber, and Elizabeth Pérez-Chiqués develop the concept of an illusion of services, demonstrating the disconnect between what the state perceives as the problem (information) and what frontline service providers and constituents perceive as the problem (structural barriers). Policies may fail not because they are poorly designed or poorly implemented, but because the policies fail to address the actual underlying problem. In the case of opioids, misplaced solutions can hide evidence of the underlying problem and exacerbate the issue that policy makers strive to fix.

The evolving terrain of opioid drug abuse renders this epidemic complex for policy and practice. While much attention has focused on opioid use among young white men in rural areas, recent estimates suggest growth in the opioid death rate among black individuals, individuals over the age of 65, and individuals who live in mid-sized metropolitan areas (Scholl et al. 2019). The collision of an evolving terrain with enduring political, regulatory, and health care structures reveals ways in which the US political process operates to yield inequities, inefficiencies, and ineffectiveness. Lessons from opioids — about racial politics, about the complexities of service delivery, about manifestations of partisan politics — extend well beyond this epidemic and reveal fundamental structural challenges embedded in US politics and policy.

Initial drafts of the articles that appear in this special issue were presented at the Politics of the Opioid Epidemic conference convened at Brown University in February 2019. The conference was supported by the Watson Institute for International and Public Affairs, the Taubman Center for American Politics and Policy, and the *Journal of Health Politics, Policy and Law*. We are grateful to Jennifer Costanza for her work organizing and implementing the conference proceedings.

References

CDC (Centers for Disease Control and Prevention). n.d. "Understanding the Epidemic." www.cdc.gov/drugoverdose/epidemic/index.html (accessed July 5, 2019).
CDC (Centers for Disease Control and Prevention). 2018. "QuickStats: Age-Adjusted Death Rates for Drug Overdose, by Race/Ethnicity — National Vital Statistics

System, United States, 2015–2016." *Morbidity and Mortality Weekly Report* 67, no. 12: 374. www.cdc.gov/mmwr/volumes/67/wr/mm6712a9.htm.

Hadland, Scott E., Ariadne Rivera-Aguirre, Brandon D. L. Marshall, and Magdalena Cerdá. 2019. "Association of Pharmaceutical Industry Marketing of Opioid Products with Mortality from Opioid-Related Overdoses." *JAMA Network Open* 2, no. 1: e186007.

Hadland, Scott E., Maxwell S. Krieger, and Brandon D. L. Marshall. 2017. "Industry Payments to Physicians Involving Opioids, 2013–2015." *American Journal of Public Health* 107, no. 9: 1493–95.

NIDA (National Institute on Drug Abuse). n.d.-a. "Overdose Death Rates." www .drugabuse.gov/related-topics/trends-statistics/overdose-death-rates (accessed August 3, 2019).

NIDA (National Institute on Drug Abuse). n.d.-b. "Opioid Overdose Crisis." www .drugabuse.gov/drugs-abuse/opioids/opioid-overdose-crisis (accessed July 7, 2019).

Scholl, Lawrence, Puja Seth, Mbabzi Kariisa, Nana Wilson, and Grant Baldwin. 2019. "Drug and Opioid-Involved Overdose Deaths, United States, 2013–2017." *Morbidity and Mortality Weekly Report* 67, no. 5152: 1419–27. www.cdc.gov/mmwr /volumes/67/wr/mm675152e1.htm (accessed August 8, 2019).

Schwartz, Robert P., Jan Gryczynski, Kevin E. O'Grady, Josh Sharfstein, Gregory Warren, Yngvild Olsen, Shannon G. Mitchell, and Jerome H. Jaffe. 2013. "Opioid Agonist Treatments and Heroin Overdose Deaths in Baltimore, Maryland, 1995–2009." *American Journal of Public Health* 103, no. 5: 917–22.

Volkow, Nora, and Francis Collins. 2017a. "The Role of Science in Addressing the Opioid Crisis." *New England Journal of Medicine* 377: 391–94.

Volkow, Nora, and Francis Collins. 2017b. "'All Scientific Hands on Deck' to End the Opioid Crisis." May 31. www.drugabuse.gov/about-nida/noras-blog/2017/05/all -scientific-hands-deck-to-end-opioid-crisis.

Walley, Alexander Y., Ziming Xuan, Maya Doe-Simkins, and Sarah Ruiz. 2013. "Opioid Overdose Rates and Implementation of Overdose Education and Nasal Naloxone Distribution in Massachusetts: Interrupted Time Series Analysis." *BMJ* 346: f174. doi.org/10.1136/bmj.f174.

Williams, John T., Susan L. Ingram, Graeme Henderson, Charles Chavkin, Mark von Zastrow, Stefan Schulz, Thomas Koch, Christopher J. Evans, and MacDonald Christie. 2013. "Regulation of μ-Opioid Receptors: Desensitization, Phosphorylation, Internalization, and Tolerance." *Pharmacological Reviews* 65, no. 1: 223–54.

Zettler, Patricia J., Margaret Foster Riley, and Aaron S. Kesselheim. 2018. "Implementing a Public Health Perspective in FDA Drug Regulation." *Food and Drug Law Journal* 73: 221–56.

Treatment versus Punishment: Understanding Racial Inequalities in Drug Policy

Jin Woo Kim
University of Pennsylvania

Evan Morgan
Brendan Nyhan
Dartmouth College

Abstract

Context: Many observers believe that the policy response to the opioid crisis is less punitive than the crack scare and that the reason is that victims are (stereotypically) white.
Methods: To assess this conjecture, we compile new longitudinal data on district-level drug-related deaths and (co)sponsorship of legislation on drug abuse in the House of Representatives over the past four decades. Using legislator fixed effects models, we then test how changes in drug-related death rates in legislators' districts predict changes in (co)sponsorship of treatment-oriented or punitive legislation in the subsequent year and assess whether these relationships vary by race of victim or drug type.
Findings: Policy makers were more likely to introduce punitive drug-related bills during the crack scare and are more likely to introduce treatment-oriented bills during the current opioid crisis. The relationship between district-level drug deaths and subsequent sponsorship of treatment-oriented legislation is greater for opioid deaths than for cocaine-related deaths and for white victims than for black victims. By contrast, district-level drug deaths are not significantly related to sponsorship of punishment-oriented bills.
Conclusions: These results suggest that the racial inequalities and double standards of drug policy still persist but in different forms.

Keywords crack, opioids, policy

The opioid crisis continues to reach new levels of severity but seemingly receives disproportionately less public attention, media coverage, and legislative action than crack cocaine did in the 1980s and 1990s. The discrepancy in responses between these two cases is not easily explained by the objective severity of the crises. More than 70,000 Americans died of drug

Journal of Health Politics, Policy and Law, Vol. 45, No. 2, April 2020
DOI 10.1215/03616878-8004850 © 2020 by Duke University Press

overdoses in 2017, a record total that far exceeds the number who died from car accidents or gun violence (Katz and Sanger-Katz 2018). Most of these deaths—47,600 (68%)—involved opioids (Scholl et al. 2018). Our analysis of the Center for Disease Control and Prevention's mortality data indicates the number of opioid-related deaths in 2016 alone (41,518) exceeds the number of cocaine-related deaths in the 1980s and 1990s combined (38,371). The scale of the opioid crisis thus outstrips any prior US drug epidemic. In addition, though the use of crack cocaine was associated with negative social and public health consequences such as increased homicides (Fryer et al. 2013; Golub and Johnson 1997), the opioid crisis has had massive social costs and has generated substantial negative externalities as well (see, e.g., Kolhatkar 2017).

As observers frequently note (e.g., Cohen 2015; Peterson and Armour 2018), the federal policy response to the opioid crisis seemingly emphasizes treatment and rehabilitation to a greater extent than the punitive approach that dominated drug policy in recent decades.[1] At the height of the crack scare, for instance, the 1992 Republican platform stated, "Drug users must face punishment, including fines and imprisonment, for contributing to the demand that makes the drug trade profitable" (Delegates to the RNC 1992). As a result of policy and administrative changes resulting from this punitive consensus, which was largely endorsed by both parties, the number of drug-related arrests and the number of people entering prison for drug crimes increased dramatically after the early 1990s (BJS 2019; Rothwell 2015). By contrast, the 2016 Republican platform highlighted how "the opioid crisis is ravaging communities all over the country, often hitting rural areas harder than urban," and called for "expeditious agreement" on a bill later signed by President Obama that sought to "expand prevention and education efforts while also promoting treatment and recovery" (CADCA 2019; Delegates to the RNC 2016). This discrepancy has frequently been noted by lawmakers and journalists, who conjecture that the shift is the result of greater empathy for stereotypically white opioid users compared to stereotypically black crack users (e.g., Glanton 2017; King 2017; Newkirk 2017).[2]

However, these conjectures about the differences between the policy response to the opioid crisis and the crack scare have not been systematically tested. In addition, little convincing evidence exists that isolates race

1. This policy difference appears to be replicated at the state level, though a comparison of drug policy across all 50 states is beyond the scope of this article. Mauer and Huling 1995 discuss changes in state approaches to drug policy during the crack scare. For recent reviews of the state policy response to the opioid crisis, see NCSL 2017 and Parker, Strunk, and Fiellin 2018.

2. Contrary to these stereotypes, the opioid crisis has claimed numerous nonwhite victims (see, e.g., Shihipar 2019).

or drug type as the key factors that explain any such differences, which could instead reflect a broader shift toward viewing drug addiction as a type of disease rather than a crime (e.g., Pew Research Center 2014).

In this article, we therefore measure the policy response to the opioid crisis in Congress and compare its content with the response to the crack scare.[3] Drawing from theory and prior research on policy responsiveness, we consider the following four research questions. First, we test whether the legislative response to the crises has differed in the aggregate, comparing the bills introduced during these epidemics and the extent to which they focus on treatment versus punishment. Second, we assess whether legislators respond to district-related drug deaths with drug policy legislation and, further, whether they respond with a treatment- or punishment-oriented approach. Third, we consider whether these patterns of responsiveness to drug deaths differ among opioids, cocaine, and methamphetamine and between white and black victims. Fourth, we test if these relationships vary over time, comparing the crack scare, the opioid crisis, and the period between them, which allows us to examine whether the recent shifts toward more empathetic approaches (if any) hold across different drug types and victims' race. Finally, we evaluate the robustness of our findings to controlling for measures of homicide deaths at the district level and test for heterogeneity in responsiveness to drug-related deaths by legislator party or factors that affect media coverage.

We evaluate these theories with newly coded data on legislative sponsorship and cosponsorship of drug-related bills in the US House of Representatives and data on drug-related deaths at the congressional district level over the past four decades. Using legislator fixed effects models, we test how changes in drug-related death rates in legislators' districts predict changes in (co)sponsorship of treatment-oriented or punitive legislation in the subsequent year and assess whether these relationships vary by race of victim or drug type. Our findings indicate that policy makers were more likely to introduce punitive drug-related bills during the crack scare and are more likely to introduce treatment-oriented bills during the current opioid crisis. We also find that legislators respond to drug deaths in their district by sponsoring more treatment-oriented legislation, but this relationship is only observed for opioid deaths and white victims. Legislators are

---

3. We focus on the federal legislative response to these drug epidemics given the nationwide attention paid to these crises and the lack of available data tracking state-level bills on drug policy across all 50 states. However, previous evidence suggests that state and federal drug policies tend to move in tandem (Mauer and Huling 1995; NCSL 2017; Parker et al. 2018). Evaluating the extent to which our findings hold at the state level is thus an important topic for future research.

specifically more responsive to opioid-related deaths than cocaine-related deaths (especially during the opioid crisis) and to white drug deaths than to black drug deaths. By contrast, we observe no evidence of a relationship between district-level drug deaths and punishment-oriented bills regardless of drug, race of victim, or era.

Theoretical Approach

What factors cause legislators to propose changes to drug policy? If political elites responded directly to objective conditions, legislative attention to the opioid crisis would be expected to be far greater than that of the crack scare. However, scholars have long emphasized that objective conditions are relevant but not decisive in setting the national agenda. Changes in issue salience often result instead from political entrepreneurs exploiting exogenous events or institutional processes to advance their policy goals (Adler and Wilkerson 2013; Kingdon and Thurber 1984). Compelling "focusing events" can also help to put issues on the policy agenda (Birkland 1997), which is shaped in part by episodic and often nonlinear changes in media coverage (Boydstun 2013; Weaver, McCombs, and Shaw 2004). By contrast, a lack of media coverage can reduce public and legislative attention to a problem and thereby reduce the likelihood of a policy response (Eisensee and Strömberg 2007).

Prior research shows that attention to the issue of illegal drugs is often divorced from objective measures of severity. In the case of crack cocaine, media coverage was extensive and frequently inaccurate (e.g., the panic over so-called crack babies; see Newkirk 2017). News reports hyped myths about crack cocaine that reinforced negative racial stereotypes (Golub and Johnson 1997)—part of a pattern of racialized news reporting that increased support for punitive approaches to crime, especially among people with negative racial attitudes (Dixon 2006; Gilliam Jr. and Iyengar 2000; Hurwitz and Peffley 1997). Politicians leveraged the increased salience of drug use to make a punishment-oriented approach to the issue an important public priority (Baumgartner and Jones 1993: 153–61). This tactic resonated with public opinion, which was heavily propunishment at the time (Enns 2014, 2016). By contrast, the opioid crisis did not center in urban areas among nonwhite Americans, lacked identifiable perpetrators like crack cocaine dealers, and came at a time when public demand for a punitive approach to crime had declined (Enns 2014, 2016). Politicians have therefore not exploited the issue as extensively as they exploited crack; similarly, media depictions have tended to be more sympathetic and less racialized (Dasgupta, Mandl, and Brownstein 2009; Harbin n.d.; Netherland and Hansen 2016).

As a result of these differences, attention to and interest in the crack scare greatly exceeded that of the opioid crisis despite the latter's far larger death toll. In 1989, a time when overdose deaths were a small fraction of the current total, 64% of Americans said drugs were the most important problem facing the country (CBS News/*New York Times* 1989). Only 2% said the same in December 2018 (Gallup 2019). Similarly, during the 1989–90 period, for example, 417 *New York Times* front-page stories mentioned crack compared with only 68 for opioids in 2017–18.[4] Public support for tough-on-crime policies has ebbed since its high-water mark in the early 1990s (Enns 2016). We therefore expect to observe a less intense and less punitive legislative response to the opioid crisis than to the crack scare. We test this expectation empirically by describing changes in treatment- and punishment-oriented legislation over the past four decades, drawing on comprehensive data of bills introduced in the US House of Representatives.

To better understand the factors that promote different responses to the two drugs, we specifically consider whether and how legislators respond to the severity of these drug epidemics in their districts. Previous research provides theoretical reasons to expect district-level responsiveness. In some cases, district conditions or characteristics may serve as a proxy for constituent preferences (Peltzman 1984). In other cases, legislators may anticipate future constituent preferences over outcomes (Canes-Wrone, Herron, and Shotts 2001) and assume they will be held accountable retrospectively (e.g., as occurred with local casualties in a war they supported—see Grose and Oppenheimer 2007). Finally, some legislators may simply seek to act on behalf of perceived constituent interests as a trustee model of representation would predict.

The available evidence, though limited, does suggest that legislators respond to district conditions and would thus be expected to respond to the severity of drug-related deaths in their districts. For instance, studies find a correspondence between district conditions and voting records on agriculture (Bellemare and Carnes 2015), poverty (Miler 2018), and free trade (Conconi, Facchini, and Zanardi 2012; Xie 2006). Further evidence

4. Results based on Nexis Uni searches for publication (*New York Times*) AND crack AND ("Section 1; Page 1" OR "Section A; Page 1" OR A1) for 1/1/1989–12/31/1990 and publication (*New York Times*) AND opioid AND ("Section 1; Page 1" OR "Section A; Page 1" OR A1) for 1/1/2017–12/31/2018.

suggests that legislators respond to changes in the status quo within their district. For instance, Winburn and Sullivan (2011) find that legislators from districts affected by Hurricane Katrina introduced more disaster relief bills after the storm, while Cayton (2017) finds that legislators from districts hardest hit by the Great Recession were more likely to vote to extend unemployment benefits.

These relationships are documented most systematically in legislative voting by Adler, Cayton, and Griffin (2018), who find that district conditions are related to voting in Congress even after accounting for constituent preferences. Similarly, Lazarus (2013) and Waggoner (2019) find that sponsorship of issue-specific legislation is strongly associated with employment levels in related industries. These relationships appear to be strongest in the House for electorally vulnerable members (Lazarus 2013), though it is important to note that such effects are typically strongly conditioned by party (see, e.g., Adler, Cayton, and Griffin 2018; Kriner and Shen 2014) and are not always observed (see in particular Fowler and Hall 2016).

There are reasons to doubt, however, that the likelihood or content of legislators' policy response to changing conditions in their districts will necessarily be proportional to the severity of the problem. First, the volume of coverage that various risks receive in the media, which has an important influence on legislative behavior (see, e.g., Arnold 2004), rarely correspond to objective measures of severity (see, e.g., Bomlitz and Brezis 2008; Frost, Frank, and Maibach 1997). Similarly, public concern tends to be driven more by cues from elites than by objective conditions—Beckett (1994) found, for instance, that the perceived importance of drugs and crime tracked with statements by government officials, not incidence rates. Finally, legislative attention tends to be driven by the strategic choices of political actors (e.g., the president and party leaders) as well as unexpected events and institutional rules and processes (Adler and Wilkerson 2013; Baumgartner and Jones 1993; Kingdon and Thurber 1984).

Representation and policy responsiveness can also be affected by organized interest group influence rather than problem severity (see, e.g., Gilens and Page 2014). For example, research shows officials elected in off-cycle elections are more likely to pursue public policy that serves the interests of organized groups (Anzia 2013) and that congressional staff members often rely on interest groups to form policy positions and gauge constituent preferences (Hertel-Fernandez, Mildenberger, and Stokes 2019).

In addition, prior work has found evidence of racial inequality in legislative responsiveness. Such inequality can take the form of direct discrimination—for example, Butler and Broockman (2011) find that white legislators are more likely to respond to emails from putatively white constituents, while minority legislators respond to putatively black constituents more often. Legislators may also differ in responsiveness to the preferences of constituents in their districts. Following the 1992 redistricting, for instance, white incumbents who lost black constituents became less responsive to black policy preferences (Overby and Cosgrove 1996). Finally, in previous research, race has consistently been found to be a significant factor in welfare policy. For example, states with higher proportions of black welfare recipients have stricter eligibility rules and offer less generous benefits (Fellowes and Rowe 2004).

We consider whether such racial inequalities exist in drug policy, a domain in which the form of elite responsiveness may depend on the stereotypical race of a drug's users or the race of the victims themselves. As noted above, negative racial stereotypes invoked by the crack scare were associated with support for punitive responses to the issues of drugs and crime (Dixon 2006; Gilliam Jr. and Iyengar 2000; Golub and Johnson 1997; Hurwitz and Peffley 1997; Newkirk 2017). As such, deaths from cocaine, especially among nonwhite victims, may be especially likely to induce a fear-oriented policy response that emphasizes punishment (Dasgupta, Mandl, and Brownstein 2009; Harbin n.d.; Netherland and Hansen 2016). By contrast, victims of the opioid crisis are seen as stereotypically white and may be viewed more sympathetically (Keller 2017; Lopez 2017; McKenzie 2017; Peterson and Armour 2018). In fact, many have claimed that the opioid crisis inspired a more treatment-oriented policy response than did the crack scare because of racial inequality in US society (e.g., Glanton 2017; King 2017; Newkirk 2017).

To empirically test these claims, we measure legislative responsiveness to drug-related deaths, evaluating whether treatment- or punishment-oriented responses vary with the drug in question and the race of the victims. This approach allows us to address the concern that the difference in legislative responses between the two drug epidemics reflects a broader shift toward viewing drug addiction as a type of disease rather than a crime (see, e.g., Pew Research Center 2014).

To better understand these relationships, we also consider legislator responsiveness to deaths from methamphetamine, a drug predominately used by whites that has generated less public sympathy than opioids but has been portrayed less negatively than crack (Cobbina 2008; Murakawa 2011). The comparison to methamphetamine will help us better understand whether policy responses to the opioid crisis have been different because its victims are stereotypically white or because they might have addictions that began with prescription drugs.

Finally, we consider two possible moderators of the relationships of interest. First, given the evidence noted above that legislative responsiveness may vary by party (e.g., Adler, Cayton, and Griffin 2018; Kriner and Shen 2014), we test whether the relationship between drug-related deaths and subsequent (co)sponsorship of treatment- or punishment-oriented legislation differs between Democrats and Republicans. Second, research shows that media coverage can have important effects on legislative behavior (e.g., Arnold 2004; Snyder and Strömberg 2010). We therefore evaluate whether variation in media coverage influences legislative responsiveness to drug-related deaths using the Snyder and Strömberg (2010) approach of exploiting district congruence with media markets, which is a plausibly exogenous source of coverage variation. We specifically test whether the relationship between drug-related deaths and legislative responsiveness varies with district/media market congruence for deaths within the district and for deaths within the media market as a whole.[5]

Data

We measure the federal legislative response to the crack scare and the opioid crisis using data for the 96th–114th Congresses (1983–2016) from the Congressional Bills Project (Adler and Wilkerson n.d.).[6] We selected every bill from this period that had been coded as pertaining to drug and alcohol abuse ("related to alcohol and illegal drug abuse, treatment, education, and health effects") or to illegal drugs ("related to illegal drug crime and enforcement [and] criminal penalties for drug crimes, including international efforts to combat drug trafficking").[7] We then further coded the summary for each qualifying bill to exclude bills solely focused on alcohol and to identify bills that contained measures addressing criminal

5. Legislators may be responsive to drug problems in nearby areas outside their district that receive news coverage and thus prompt fears among their constituents.

6. The Congressional Bills Project labels bill summaries according to the topic coding system of the Policy Agendas Project (PAP). The PAP codebook is available at www.comparative agendas.net/pages/master-codebook.

7. These PAP categories include bills addressing illegal drugs as well as those addressing abuse of prescription drugs. To ensure that we did not miss a substantial number of opioid-related bills related to legal prescription drugs, we searched the categories of bills "related to prescription drug coverage, programs to pay for prescription drugs, and policy to reduce the cost of prescription drugs" or "related to the regulation and promotion of pharmaceuticals, medical devices, and clinical labs" for the keywords pain, opioid, addict, and substance. These returned only 67 cases during a 44-year study period (1983–2016). We therefore did not include them in our analyses.

or civil penalties or promoting prevention, treatment, and rehabilitation (34 of the bills, or 2.3%, do both).[8] We then merge information on these bills with cosponsorship data from GovTrack.[9]

From these measures, we construct four simple binary measures of bill sponsorship and cosponsorship for each member of the House of Representatives from 1983 to 2016 at the year level.[10] Specifically, for each member of Congress, we measure whether they sponsored at least one prevention- or treatment-oriented bill related to drug abuse ("treatment bill") and whether they sponsored at least one punishment-oriented bill related to drugs ("punishment bill").[11] We then construct analogous measures for legislative cosponsorship, a symbolic but consequential act in which legislators officially indicate their support for a bill that another legislator has sponsored (Koger 2003).

Our primary independent variables are drug-related death rates by year at the congressional district level. To obtain these, we analyze confidential multiple cause of death data from the Division of Vital Statistics at the National Center for Health Statistics. These data provide individual-level records on the causes of death and contributing conditions for every American who dies in a given year. We identify the causes of death for each variable using ICD-9 and ICD-10 codes, which are provided for each death in the data. Following standard practices in the literature, we use a combination of diagnosis and external cause codes (ICD-9) and multiple cause of death codes (ICD-10) to identify cocaine-, opioid-, and methamphetamine-related deaths.[12] We specifically calculate the total number of drug poisoning deaths overall and separately for whites, blacks,

8. We sought to specifically identify bills that increased penalties for illegal drug use or drug abuse. We therefore excluded bills whose summaries specifically mentioned reducing penalties or specifically targeted drug distributors. Intercoder reliability ratings for the codings we employed in this study exceeded conventional norms in blind tests using randomized samples of bills. Results and detailed coding rules are provided in the online-only appendix.

9. The source is James H. Fowler, Andrew Scott Waugh, and Yunkyu Sohn, "Cosponsorship Network Data," jhfowler.ucsd.edu/cosponsorship.htm (accessed October 18, 2019).

10. We consider the set of legislators who served in each Congress during this period with data from the Legislative Effectiveness Project (Volden and Wiseman 2014). Each is considered to serve in both years except for those who left office in the first year of a given Congress because they died, resigned, etc. or entered office in the second year via appointment, special election, etc. (data from Stewart and Woon n.d.; Swift et al. 2000). We follow standard practice in the Congress literature and treat party switchers as new members after a switch and apply analogous year-level exclusions depending on the switch's timing.

11. We use binary measures due to concerns about skew in a small number of variables for the outcome measures and the greater robustness of ordinary least squares (Angrist and Pischke 2009).

12. See the online-only appendix for a detailed list of our coding rules. We note in particular that we observe no evidence of discontinuities in the aggregate time series of overall or drug-specific deaths during the switch from ICD-9 to ICD-10 in 1999 (see fig. 1). We thus pool the data over the study period.

and people from other racial/ethnic groups. We also calculate the total number of deaths related to opioids, cocaine, and methamphetamines. Finally, we calculate the total number of homicide deaths. We then aggregate these county-level totals, which are based on the location of the deceased's residence, by year at the congressional district level and divide them by the district population, transforming them into drug-related death rates.[13]

To consider the role of media coverage in political responsiveness to drug-related deaths, we construct two measures. First, because legislators might respond to media coverage of drug deaths outside of their district, we estimate drug-related death rates at the media market level using data from Gentzkow and Shapiro (2008). In addition, we use the Snyder and Strömberg (2010) measures of congruence between media markets and congressional districts to identify plausibly exogenous variation in coverage intensity that might affect legislator responsiveness to drug-related deaths in their district.

Results

We first present descriptive graphs and statistics for our primary independent and dependent variables, illustrating how drug death rates and legislative policy approaches to drug abuse have varied over our study period.[14] Figure 1 plots annual drug-related death rates by year for all drugs and for opioids and cocaine over the 1983–2016 period. As the figure indicates, drug-related death rates climbed modestly from 1983 to the early 2000s before accelerating in recent years, pushing the mortality rate to .19 per 1,000 people in 2016. This increase was largely driven by opioids. During the crack scare (1983–95), opioids and cocaine were associated with a nearly identical number of deaths despite widespread public and media attention to crack cocaine. Death rates from opioids began to outstrip cocaine death rates in the mid-1990s, however, rising from .02 per 1,000 people in 1995 to .13 per 1,000 in 2016. Opioids now kill far more Americans per year than all drugs did at the crack scare's peak.[15]

---

13. When counties were split across more than one congressional district, we allocated deaths proportionally with population weights from the most recent census, which covers the 98th Congress and later. We used redistricting data from Carson et al. 2007 to map congressional districts prior to the 1980 census redistricting to counties. We were not able to map 27 districts from this period to counties and thus restricted our main analyses to 1983 and later (results are very similar when including 1979–1982; available upon request).

14. Table A2 in the online-only appendix provides descriptive statistics of the key variables.

15. See figure A1 in the online-only appendix for corresponding race-specific death rates per 1,000 Americans.

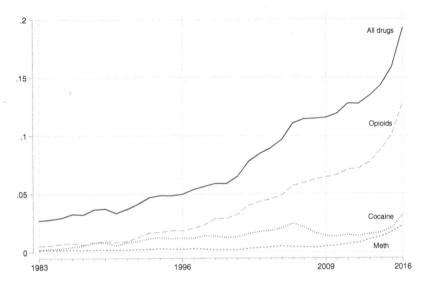

Figure 1 Yearly drug-related death rates (per 1,000 people).

Notes: Total drug-related deaths per year from all illegal drugs and from opioids, metham-phetamines, and cocaine. Calculated with data from the National Center for Health Statistics (see the online-only appendix for coding details).

To understand how policy approaches to drug abuse vary over this time period, figure 2 presents smoothed models of over-time variation in legislative policy approaches to drugs. These estimates start in 1979 to show pre-study period trends and avoid extrapolation in the local polynomial fits. The figure shows lawmakers introduced more drug-related bills during the crack scare than later on. When compared with figure 1, which shows that far more people have died of drug poisoning in recent years, this figure demonstrates a striking lack of correspondence between drug mortality and policy responses.[16] While the figure shows that the number of drug-related bills has been increasing during the opioid crisis, the total is still less than in the mid-1980s. These data also indicate that legislators were more likely to sponsor bills that proposed a punishment-oriented approach to drug abuse and addiction than a treatment-oriented approach during the crack scare of 1983–95.[17] This differential was no longer consistently

16. For example, the total number of bills sponsored decreased in the mid-1990s despite the fact that neither cocaine deaths nor overall drug deaths decreased during that period. This decline is likely linked to the decline in media attention to the crack scare around that time (Hartman and Golub 1999).

17. The smoothed year-level estimates in these graphs range from 0 to 0.03, but the yearly data vary from 0.01 to 0.07 for punishment bills (1989, when 30 members [7%] introduced bills) and from 0 to 0.04 for treatment bills (1991, when 16 members [4%] introduced bills).

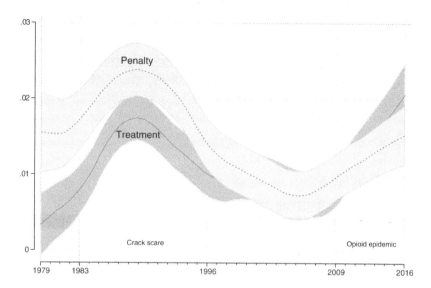

Figure 2 Drug abuse bill sponsorship rates by policy approach.

Notes: Outcome is a yearly binary indicator of sponsorship of one or more bills related to treatment or punishment of drug abuse among members of the House of Representatives (local polynomial fits with bandwidth of three years). Data from the Congressional Bills Project (Adler and Wilkerson n.d.).

measurable after 1995. Indeed, the number of treatment bills has been growing more rapidly than punishment bills since the beginning of the opioid crisis, and the mid-2010s represent the first time that treatment-oriented policy responses became more prevalent than penalty-oriented ones in our data.

Next, we estimate a series of ordinary least squares (OLS) models to evaluate our theoretical expectations. Each model predicts legislative bill (co)sponsorship using drug-related death rates in a legislator's House district. We calculate separate measures by drug type (total drug-related deaths, opioid deaths, and cocaine deaths) and by race of victim (white or black).[18] Each death rate measure is calculated as the total number of deaths per 1,000 district residents and lagged by one year to ensure a plausible temporal relationship between deaths and bill sponsorship.[19] These models include legislator fixed effects to account for time-invariant

18. In this study we focus specifically on white deaths, because they are the majority racial group at the national level, and black deaths, because they are the group critics argue have been treated the worst in drug policy.

19. We normalize by district population to ensure the death rate measures are comparable across districts.

factors such as party that might induce a spurious relationship between drug deaths and (co)sponsorship of drug-related bills.[20] We use legislator fixed effects rather than district fixed effects because districts change over time due to redistricting, and legislators tend to behave quite consistently (see, e.g., Poole and Rosenthal 2007). These fixed effects account for all baseline differences among legislators, allowing us to capture how changes in drug death rates in each legislator's district predicts changes in his or her drug policy responses in the coming year. It is therefore not necessary to control for legislator party or other time-invariant characteristics. We also include fixed effects by census region-year to account for correlated temporal shocks (possibly region specific) that do not vary across legislators or districts and could produce spurious relationships such as changes in national drug policy, differences in the availability of different kinds of drugs over time such as fentanyl, and the growth in support for criminal justice reform in recent years. These fixed effects also account for any (linear or nonlinear) national trends that are correlated across districts. Finally, we separately cluster the standard errors by legislator and region-year to account for any remaining within-legislator or within-region-year correlation (e.g., legislators reintroducing bills they have sponsored repeatedly over time). These fixed effects models are identified using temporal variation in drug-related deaths within (not between) legislators, which we take as exogenous. Per Mummolo and Peterson (2018), we present summary statistics for this identifying within-district variation in table A3 in the online-only appendix.

We begin our analysis by estimating the relationship between district drug-related deaths and subsequent sponsorship and cosponsorship of treatment-oriented bills (tables 1a and 1b, respectively). Our results indicate that drug-related deaths are significantly positively associated with subsequent legislative sponsorship of treatment-oriented bills ($p < .05$; column 1 of table 1a). However, this pattern of responsiveness to drug deaths varies by drug type and victim race. We find that opioid deaths are significantly associated with subsequent sponsorship of treatment-oriented legislation ($p < .01$ in column 2, $p < .005$ in column 5) but cocaine and methamphetamine deaths are not (columns 3 and 4). Similarly, deaths of white drug victims are positively associated with subsequent treatment bills ($p < .005$; columns 6 and 8). By contrast, deaths of black victims are

20. The key identifying assumption of a fixed effects model is that a confounding variable does not vary over time. This assumption would not hold if changes in crime rates are correlated with both drug severity and policy responses. We address this concern below by showing that our results are robust for controlling for district-level homicide rates.

Table 1 Sponsorship/Cosponsorship of Treatment-Oriented Bills by Prior Drug Deaths

(a) Sponsorship of Treatment-Oriented Bills

	(1)	(2)	(3)	(4)	(5)	(6)	(7)	(8)
Total drug deaths	0.196* (0.078)							
Opioid deaths		0.296** (0.112)			0.432*** (0.135)			
Cocaine deaths			−0.055 (0.265)		−0.683* (0.334)			
Meth deaths				0.853 (0.476)	0.567 (0.472)			
White drug deaths						0.274*** (0.082)		0.327*** (0.080)
Black drug deaths							−0.371 (0.249)	−0.690* (0.283)
Legislator fixed effects	Y	Y	Y	Y	Y	Y	Y	Y
Region-year fixed effects	Y	Y	Y	Y	Y	Y	Y	Y
Legislators	1243	1243	1243	1243	1243	1243	1243	1243
Total N	13008	13008	13008	13008	13008	13008	13008	13008

Table 1 (*continued*)

(b) Cosponsorship of Treatment-Oriented Bills

	(1)	(2)	(3)	(4)	(5)	(6)	(7)	(8)
Total drug deaths	0.096 (0.214)							
Opioid deaths		0.560* (0.237)			1.050*** (0.264)			
Cocaine deaths			−0.655 (0.553)		−2.090*** (0.680)			
Meth deaths				−0.652 (1.008)	−1.250 (0.994)			
White drug deaths						0.170 (0.244)		0.230 (0.244)
Black drug deaths							−0.561 (0.661)	−0.786 (0.685)
Legislator fixed effects	Y	Y	Y	Y	Y	Y	Y	Y
Region-year fixed effects	Y	Y	Y	Y	Y	Y	Y	Y
Legislators	1243	1243	1243	1243	1243	1243	1243	1243
Total N	13003	13003	13003	13003	13003	13003	13003	13003

* $p < 0.05$, ** $p < .01$, *** $p < .005$ (two-sided p values); OLS models with two-way clustering by legislator and region-year (Cameron, Gelbach, and Miller 2011; Correia 2016). Constant is suppressed. Outcome variables are a binary measure of legislative sponsorship or cosponsorship of one or more bills related to treatment of drug use among members of the House of Representatives during the 1983–2016 period. All drug-related death variables are calculated from mortality records as deaths per 1,000 district residents and are lagged by one year.

negatively associated with treatment legislation when entered into the same model as deaths of white victims (p < .05; column 8), though we cannot be certain that this negative coefficient reflects a causal relationship.[21] Importantly, we can reject the nulls of no difference between the effects of opioid- and cocaine-related deaths (p < .05; column 4) and between the effects of deaths of white and black victims (p < .005; column 7). We observe a similar pattern in table 1b of differential responsiveness in cosponsorship of treatment-oriented bills to opioid- and cocaine-related deaths (p < .005; column 5), though we find no measurable difference by victim race (column 8).

To interpret the magnitude of these relationships, it is important to note first that the base rate of treatment-oriented drug bill sponsorship is only 1.6%. We must also consider the range of variation in white drug deaths accounting for legislator and region-year fixed effects (Mummolo and Peterson 2018). If white drug deaths increased by two standard deviations, the expected increase in the likelihood of treatment bill sponsorship using the results from column 6 of table 1a is 1.04 percentage points, which represents an increase of 83% in relative terms from the treatment bill sponsorship base rate of 1.26%.[22] An analogous increase of two standard deviations in within-district opioid deaths would generate a 1.24 percentage point increase in the likelihood of treatment bill sponsorship (a 98% increase in relative terms).

The patterns of differential treatment-oriented responses to drug deaths by victim race (table 1a) and type of drug (table 1b) that we describe above do not clearly hold for punishment-oriented bills, however. Table 2a shows no significant association between prior-year drug deaths and sponsorship of punishment-oriented bills regardless of whether we consider total drug deaths (column 1) or disaggregate them by type of drug (columns 2–4) or race of victim (columns 5–7). We therefore do not find evidence that objective conditions at the local level affect the decision to sponsor such bills (unlike the relationship we observe at the national level, which is presented in figure 2). Interestingly, in table 2b, we do observe evidence that legislators are more responsive in cosponsoring punishment-oriented legislation as opioid deaths and white drug deaths increase (columns 5 and 8), which is somewhat inconsistent with our theoretical expectation. Taken together with table 1, this finding suggests that representatives may be

21. The negative association is statistically significant in the model for controlling for white victims (p < .05; column 8) but not in the bivariate model (column 7). We therefore cannot rule out the possibility that the column 8 estimate reflects posttreatment bias (the same factors causing black deaths may also be causing white deaths).

22. Such an increase would, if generalized, translate into more than five additional bills that year across 435 House members.

Table 2 Sponsorship/Cosponsorship of Punishment-Oriented Bills by Prior Drug Deaths

(a) Sponsorship of Punishment-Oriented Bills

	(1)	(2)	(3)	(4)	(5)	(6)	(7)	(8)
Total drug deaths	-0.039							
	(0.067)							
Opioid deaths		-0.077			0.009			
		(0.070)			(0.085)			
Cocaine deaths			-0.389		-0.406			
			(0.362)		(0.437)			
Meth deaths				0.032	0.113			
				(0.397)	(0.408)			
White drug deaths						-0.045		-0.044
						(0.056)		(0.045)
Black drug deaths							-0.060	-0.017
							(0.432)	(0.427)
Legislator fixed effects	Y	Y	Y	Y	Y	Y	Y	Y
Region-year fixed effcts	Y	Y	Y	Y	Y	Y	Y	Y
Legislators	1243	1243	1243	1243	1243	1243	1243	1243
Total N	13003	13003	13003	13003	13003	13003	13003	13003

(continued)

Table 2 Sponsorship/Cosponsorship of Punishment-Oriented Bills by Prior Drug Deaths (*continued*)

(b) Cosponsorship of Punishment-Oriented Bills

	(1)	(2)	(3)	(4)	(5)	(6)	(7)	(8)
Total drug deaths	0.307* (0.139)							
Opioid deaths		0.637** (0.162)			0.820** (0.224)			
Cocaine deaths			0.366 (0.521)		-0.767 (0.676)			
Meth deaths				0.049 (1.189)	-0.611 (1.186)			
White drug deaths						0.375* (0.152)		0.403** (0.154)
Black drug deaths							0.035 (0.587)	-0.358 (0.616)
Legislator fixed effects	Y	Y	Y	Y	Y	Y	Y	Y
Region-year fixed effects	Y	Y	Y	Y	Y	Y	Y	Y
Legislators	1243	1243	1243	1243	1243	1243	1243	1243
Total N	13003	13003	13003	13003	13003	13003	13003	13003

* p < 0.05, ** p < .01, *** p < .005 (two-sided p values); OLS models with two-way clustering by legislator and region-year (Cameron, Gelbach, and Miller 2011; Correia 2016). Constant is suppressed. Outcome variables are a binary measure of legislative sponsorship (table 2a) or cosponsorship (table 2b) of one or more bills related to punishment of drug abuse among members of the House of Representatives during the 1983–2016 period. All drug-related death variables are calculated from mortality records as deaths per 1,000 district residents and are lagged by one year.

willing to respond to or address opioid deaths and white deaths using punitive as well as treatment-oriented approaches. However, this conclusion must be treated as tentative—unlike in table 1, we cannot reject the null of no difference in effects with cocaine deaths and black drug deaths, respectively.

Broadly, these results suggest that district-level drug deaths increase the (co)sponsorship of treatment-oriented bills, especially for opioid overdoses and when the victims are white, but do not have a strong or consistent effect on punishment-oriented bills. In tables 3 and A4, we examine the extent to which this pattern varies over time. To do so, we estimate versions of previous models predicting sponsorship of treatment- or punishment-oriented bills in which we interact drug deaths with indicators for the crack era, which we define as 1983–95, and the opioid era, which we define as 2009–16.[23] The coefficients on the interaction terms test whether these relationships vary by era compared to the reference period of 1996–2008.

We first consider differences over time in responsiveness to drug deaths with sponsorship of treatment-oriented bills. Consistent with our expectation, table 3 indicates that legislators respond to drug deaths in the opioid era with treatment-oriented legislation ($p < .05$ for the marginal effect in the 2009–16 period), though we cannot reject the null of no difference in effects with the other two eras (column 1). The story becomes clearer when we focus specifically on deaths by drug type. The fully specified model considering opioid, cocaine, and methamphetamine deaths (column 5) shows that legislators sponsored more treatment bills as opioid deaths increased in their district in the interim period (1996–2008; $p < .01$) and especially during the opioid crisis (2009–16 marginal effect; $p < .005$). As a result, we can reject the null of no difference in the relationship between opioid and cocaine deaths only during the opioid crisis ($p < .05$). We also find that white drug deaths were significantly associated with treatment bill sponsorship in the interim period and during the opioid crisis, but not during the crack era (columns 6 and 8). Moreover, this relationship is significantly different from the one observed for black drug deaths in the interim period and opioid crisis ($p < .005$).

For ease of understanding, we plot the relationship between drug deaths and treatment bills by era in figure 3 (based on columns 1–4 and 6–7 of table 3). It shows that the relationship between drug deaths and treatment-oriented bills has become stronger overall (figure 3a). However, this finding

23. By 2009 opioid overuse had become a sufficient enough concern that the Federal Drug Administration launched its Safe Use Initiative (FDA 2019). Heroin deaths started to rise in 2011, and synthetic opioid deaths began to increase in 2014 (Ciccarone 2019).

Table 3 Sponsorship of Treatment-Oriented Drugs Bills by Time Period and Prior Drug Deaths

	(1)	(2)	(3)	(4)	(5)	(6)	(7)	(8)
Total drug deaths	0.106*							
	(0.050)							
Total × crack era	0.044							
	(0.096)							
Total × opioid era	0.162							
	(0.098)							
Opioid deaths		0.099			0.251**			
		(0.077)			(0.093)			
Opioid × crack era		0.108			−0.289			
		(0.296)			(0.300)			
Opioid × opioid era		0.316*			0.338*			
		(0.127)			(0.148)			
Cocaine deaths			−0.221		−0.603			
			(0.258)		(0.329)			
Cocaine × crack era			0.433		0.713			
			(0.361)		(0.416)			
Cocaine × opioid era			0.256		−0.639			
			(0.348)		(0.407)			
Meth deaths				0.202	0.187			
				(0.479)	(0.499)			
Meth × crack era				0.011	0.128			
				(0.961)	(0.962)			

Table 3 (continued)

	(1)	(2)	(3)	(4)	(5)	(6)	(7)	(8)
Meth×opioid era				1.085*	0.550			
				(0.534)	(0.595)			
White drug deaths						0.193***		0.245***
						(0.055)		(0.059)
White×crack era						-0.053		-0.174
						(0.143)		(0.178)
White×opioid era						0.140		0.135
						(0.102)		(0.100)
Black drug deaths							-0.517	-0.803**
							(0.272)	(0.306)
Black×crack era							0.569*	0.639
							(0.281)	(0.339)
Black×opioid era							-0.150	-0.109
							(0.209)	(0.215)
Legislator fixed effects	Y	Y	Y	Y	Y	Y	Y	Y
Region-year fixed effects	Y	Y	Y	Y	Y	Y	Y	Y
Legislators	1243	1243	1243	1243	1243	1243	1243	1243
Total N	13003	13003	13003	13003	13003	13003	13003	13003

* $p < 0.05$, ** $p < .01$, *** $p < .005$ (two-sided p values); OLS models with two-way clustering by legislator and region-year (Cameron, Gelbach, and Miller 2011; Correia 2016). Constant is suppressed. Outcome is a binary measure of legislative sponsorship of one or more treatment-oriented bills related to drug abuse or illegal drugs among members of the House of Representatives during the 1983–2016 period. All drug-related death variables are calculated from mortality records as deaths per 1,000 district residents and are lagged by one year. The crack era is defined as 1983–95 and the opioid era as 2009–16 (reference category is 1996–2008).

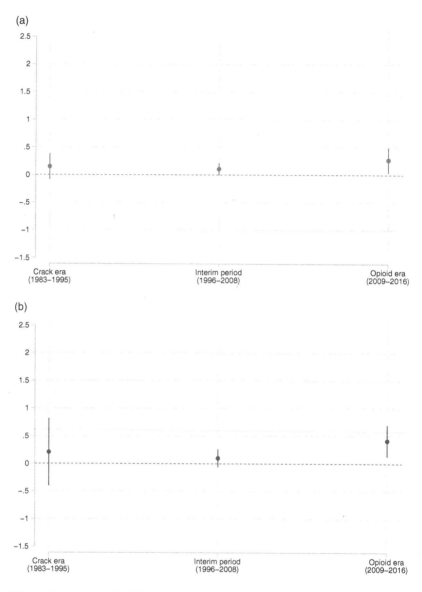

Figure 3 Marginal effects of drug deaths on treatment sponsorship by drug type/race of victim: (a) all drugs; (b) opioids; (c) cocaine; (d) methamphetamine; (e) white victims; (f) black victims.

Notes: Marginal effects of drug deaths on sponsorship of one or more bills related to treatment of drug use among members of the House of Representatives. Figures 3a, 3b, 3c, and 3d correspond to models 1, 2, 3, and 4 in table 3. Figures 3e and 3f correspond to models 6 and 7 in table 3. All drug-related death variables are calculated from mortality records as deaths per 1,000 district residents and are lagged by one year (see the online-only appendix for coding details). Data from the Congressional Bills Project (Adler and Wilkerson n.d.).

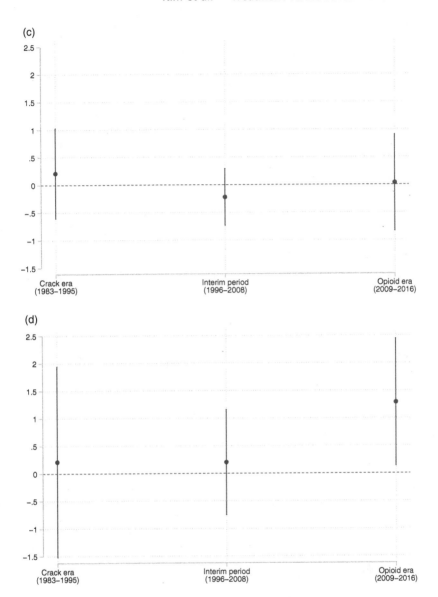

Figure 3   (continued)

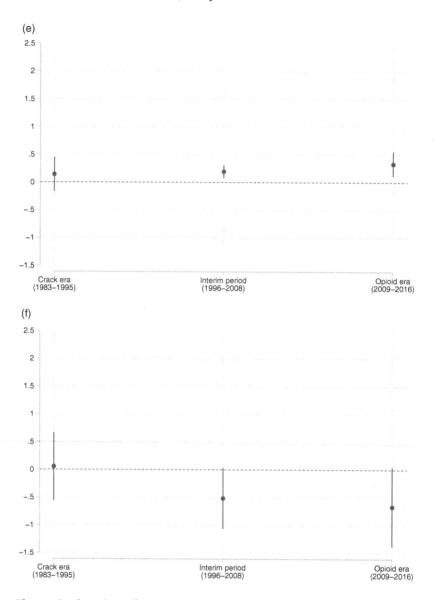

Figure 3   (continued)

holds for opioid-related deaths (figure 3b) and methamphetamine-related deaths (figure 3d), but not those related to cocaine (figure 3c), which are not estimated precisely. The shift over time toward treatment-oriented responses seems to be driven by drugs that are believed to have most affected white communities.[24]

Similarly, there is a noticeable difference in treatment policy responses to drug deaths by victim race. Specifically, legislators are responsive to the deaths of white victims (figure 3e) and not to black victims (figure 3f)—a racial gap in treatment-related drug policy that is widest during the current opioid crisis.

None of the relationships we describe above are observed for punishment-oriented bills, however (table A4). We find no significant association between prior-year drug deaths and bill sponsorship in any era for any measure. These results suggest that sponsorship of punishment-oriented bills is not a response to the local severity of drug use (legislators may instead be responding to other factors such as media coverage or public opinion).

We next consider the robustness of our results. The most plausible threat to our design is that changes in drug deaths are correlated with other crimes and that our models pick up the effects of these non-drug-related crimes. To address this concern, we calculate homicide rates at the district level (the measure of crime incidence that is most consistently measured across districts) and replicate all the models reported in the text above with this measure as a control variable. Our results, which are reported in tables A5–A8 of the online-only appendix, are very similar to those discussed above.

Finally, we consider two possible moderators of the relationships we observe—political parties and media coverage. We first estimate whether the relationship between district-related drug deaths and sponsorship of treatment- or punishment-oriented legislation varies by party identification. Tables A9 and A10 in the online-only appendix show, however, that we cannot reject the null hypothesis of no difference in responsiveness (i.e., the relationship between district-level drug deaths and bill sponsorship) between Democrats and Republicans across all the measures of drug-related deaths considered above (i.e., by race and drug type). Similarly, we observe little consistent evidence that the relationship between drug deaths and legislative responsiveness varies by congruence between media markets and congressional district boundaries (tables A11–A12). Finally, responsiveness to deaths at the media market level is similar to deaths at

---

24. The estimated marginal effect size is larger for methamphetamines, which likely reflects the reduced level of within-legislator variation in deaths compared to opioids.

the district level (table A13) but these relationships again do not measurably vary by congruence (tables A14–A15), providing little convincing evidence that media coverage drives responsiveness.

Conclusion

The opioid crisis has sparked a public debate over how policy makers have addressed drug abuse in recent decades. Many have suggested that policy responses to the opioid crisis emphasize treatment and have speculated that race explains the changes (e.g., Peterson and Armour 2018), but lack convincing evidence for this claim. Our study provides the first systematic comparison of the federal legislative policy response to the crack scare and the opioid crisis. Despite the massive increase in opioid overdose deaths since 2009, legislators were more likely to sponsor legislation related to drugs during the crack scare. However, we do find that members of Congress have responded to the opioid crisis by proposing more treatment-oriented policies. We focus specifically on legislator responsiveness to local drug deaths, which we find varies by type of drug and race of victim (but not legislator party or factors that affect media coverage). Policy makers appear to respond to district-level drug mortality by increasing the likelihood that they propose treatment-oriented legislation, but this response is driven by responsiveness to victims of opioid overdoses (especially in recent years) and to white drug deaths. Punitive drug policies, by contrast, seem to be unrelated to district-level mortality rates. These results suggest that the political system is differentially sensitive to the suffering of white victims of the opioid crisis and is unusually willing to offer treatment-oriented policies on their behalf.

Importantly, the differential responsiveness by race found in this study is consistent with previous research that has documented various forms of racial discrimination in political representation (e.g., Butler and Broockman 2011; Overby and Cosgrove 1996). Our study contributes to research on the interaction of race and representation by showing how urgent problems such as drug epidemics can generate unequal policy responses depending on which racial groups are affected. Similar forms of double standards and differential treatment likely exist in other issue domains such as welfare or criminal justice (see, e.g., Fellowes and Rowe 2004), though more research is needed to better understand the objective conditions of black and white communities and to compare legislative responses to those conditions. Further research is also needed to determine how to most effectively improve representation for disadvantaged communities and mitigate these inequalities.

Of course, this study has limitations that should be noted. First, we do not consider congressional voting, constituent service, floor speeches, or other forms of potential legislative responsiveness to district conditions. Second, we focus on legislative responsiveness to drug-related deaths, not other harms from drug use. Our reliance on mortality data necessarily highlights opioids due to the greater likelihood of lethal overdoses from its use (especially with synthetic opioids like fentanyl). These data also span the 1999 transition from ICD-9 to ICD-10 cause of death codes, which may reduce the comparability of data between the crack scare and the opioid crisis (though we observe no evidence of discontinuities). Third, future research should seek to extend this approach to study drug policy responsiveness in the states, which plays a critical role in both criminal justice and public health policy under the US federal system. It would also be valuable to examine variation in responses by prosecutors, judges, public health agencies, and other federal and state actors to local-level drug mortality during the opioid crisis. Finally, scholars should devote further attention to possible changes over time in the content of media coverage of drug use, a possible mechanism of support for treatment-oriented policies (e.g., Harbin n.d.).

Still, this study represents an important step toward understanding the forces shaping the policy response to one of the most important issues in contemporary US politics. Given the staggering human toll of the opioid crisis, the stakes could hardly be higher.

■ ■ ■

Jin Woo Kim is a George Gerbner postdoctoral fellow at the Annenberg School for Communication at the University of Pennsylvania. His research examines the effects of political information on public opinion.

Evan Morgan is a data engineer at Mastercard. As an undergraduate at Dartmouth College, he studied the intersection of public policy and the opioid crisis.

Brendan Nyhan is professor of government at Dartmouth College. His research, which focuses on misperceptions about politics and health care, has been published in journals such as the *American Journal of Political Science*, *Journal of Politics*, and *Pediatrics*. He previously served as a Robert Wood Johnson scholar in health policy research and professor of public policy at the University of Michigan. Nyhan is also a contributor to The Upshot at the *New York Times* and GEN, the politics site from Medium; cofounder of Bright Line Watch, a watchdog group monitoring the state of US democracy; and a 2018 Andrew Carnegie fellow.
nyhan@dartmouth.edu

Acknowledgments

We thank Jack Davidson and Lucas Maiman for outstanding research assistance and Devin Caughey, Mia Costa, Jesse Crosson, Alexander Furnas, Sarah Gollust, Gregory Koger, Josh McCrain, Andrew Reeves, Christopher Warshaw, and participants in the Politics of the Opioid Epidemic conference at Brown University for helpful comments. We are also grateful to the Congressional Bills Project, the Legislative Effectiveness Project, and the National Center for Health Statistics for providing the data used in our analysis, and to the Stamps Family Charitable Foundation and the Dartmouth Politics and Law Program for supporting Morgan's work on the project. Finally, we are grateful to our colleague D. J. Flynn, who helped conceive the article and code the legislative bills data.

References

Adler, E. Scott, Adam F. Cayton, and John D. Griffin. 2018. "Representation When Constituent Opinion and District Conditions Collide." *Political Research Quarterly* 71, no. 3: 681–94.

Adler, E. Scott, and John Wilkerson. n.d. "Congressional Bills Project: 1979–2014." congressionalbills.org/download.html (accessed January 14, 2020).

Adler, E. Scott, and John D. Wilkerson. 2013. *Congress and the Politics of Problem Solving*. Cambridge: Cambridge University Press.

Angrist, Joshua D., and Jörn-Steffen Pischke. 2009. *Mostly Harmless Econometrics: An Empiricist's Companion*. Princeton, NJ: Princeton University Press.

Anzia, Sarah F. 2013. *Timing and Turnout: How Off-Cycle Elections Favor Organized Groups*. Chicago: University of Chicago Press.

Arnold, R. Douglas. 2004. *Congress, the Press, and Political Accountability*. Princeton, NJ: Princeton University Press.

Baumgartner, Frank R., and Brian D. Jones. 1993. *Agendas and Instability in American Politics*. Chicago: University of Chicago Press.

Beckett, Katherine. 1994. "Setting the Public Agenda: 'Street Crime' and Drug Use in American Politics." *Social Problems* 41, no. 3: 425–47.

Bellemare, Marc F., and Nicholas Carnes. 2015. "Why Do Members of Congress Support Agricultural Protection?" *Food Policy* 50: 20–34. doi.org/10.1016/j.foodpol.2014.10.010.

BJS (Bureau of Justice Statistics). 2019. "Drugs and Crime Facts." www.bjs.gov/content/dcf/enforce.cfm (accessed January 11, 2019).

Birkland, Thomas A. 1997. *After Disaster: Agenda Setting, Public Policy, and Focusing Events*. Washington, DC: Georgetown University Press.

Bomlitz, Larisa J., and Mayer Brezis. 2008. "Misrepresentation of Health Risks by Mass Media." *Journal of Public Health* 30, no. 2: 202–4.

Boydstun, Amber E. 2013. *Making the News: Politics, the Media, and Agenda Setting*. Chicago: University of Chicago Press.

Butler, Daniel M., and David E. Broockman. 2011. "Do Politicians Racially Discriminate against Constituents? A Field Experiment on State Legislators." *American Journal of Political Science* 55, no. 3: 463–77.

CADCA (Community Anti-Drug Coalitions of America). n.d. "The Comprehensive Addiction and Recovery Act (CARA)." www.cadca.org/comprehensive-addiction -and-recovery-act-cara (accessed January 11, 2019).

Cameron, A. Colin, Jonah B. Gelbach, and Douglas L. Miller. 2011. "Robust Inference with Multiway Clustering." *Journal of Business and Economic Statistics* 29, no. 2: 238–49.

Canes-Wrone, Brandice, Michael C. Herron, and Kenneth W. Shotts. 2001. "Leadership and Pandering: A Theory of Executive Policymaking." *American Journal of Political Science* 45, no. 3: 532–50.

Carson, Jamie L., Michael H. Crespin, Charles J. Finocchiaro, and David W. Rohde. 2007. "Redistricting and Party Polarization in the US House of Representatives." *American Politics Research* 35, no. 6: 878–904.

Cayton, Adam F. 2017. "Consistency versus Responsiveness: Do Members of Congress Change Positions on Specific Issues in Response to Their Districts?" *Political Research Quarterly* 70, no. 1: 3–18.

CBS News/*New York Times*. 1989. "CBS News/*New York Times* Drug Poll, September 1989." USCBSNYT.091189.R02. CBS News/New York Times (producer). Cornell University, Ithaca, NY: Roper Center for Public Opinion Research, iPOLL (distributor; accessed January 11, 2019).

Ciccarone, Daniel. 2019. "The Triple Wave Epidemic: Supply and Demand Drivers of the US Opioid Overdose Crisis." *International Journal on Drug Policy*, February 1. doi.org/10.1016/j.drugpo.2019.01.010.

Cobbina, Jennifer E. 2008. "Race and Class Differences in Print Media Portrayals of Crack Cocaine and Methamphetamine." *Journal of Criminal Justice and Popular Culture* 15, no. 2: 145–67.

Cohen, Andrew. 2015. "How White Users Made Heroin a Public-Health Problem." *Atlantic*, August 12. theatlantic.com/politics/archive/2015/08/crack/heroin-and -race/401015/.

Conconi, Paola, Giovanni Facchini, and Maurizio Zanardi. 2012. "Fast-Track Authority and International Trade Negotiations." *American Economic Journal: Economic Policy* 4, no. 3: 146–89.

Correia, Sergio. 2017. "Linear Models with High-Dimensional Fixed Effects: An Efficient and Feasible Estimator." Working paper. scorreia.com/research/hdfe.pdf (accessed October 18, 2019).

Dasgupta, Nabarun, Kenneth D. Mandl, and John S. Brownstein. 2009. "Breaking the News or Fueling the Epidemic? Temporal Association between News Media Report Volume and Opioid-Related Mortality." *PloS One* 4, no. 11: e7758.

Delegates to the RNC. 1992. "The Vision Shared: The Republican Platform, Uniting Our Family, Our Country, Our World." Republican Party Platforms, the American President Project, University of California, Santa Cruz. www.presidency.ucsb.edu /documents/republican-party-platform-1992 (accessed January 11, 2019).

Delegates to the RNC. 2016. "Restoring the American Dream." Republican Party Platforms, the American President Project, University of California, Santa Cruz. www.presidency.ucsb.edu/documents/2016-republican-party-platform (accessed January 11, 2019).

Dixon, Travis L. 2006. "Psychological Reactions to Crime News Portrayals of Black Criminals: Understanding the Moderating Roles of Prior News Viewing and Stereotype Endorsement." *Communication Monographs* 73, no. 2: 162–87.

Eisensee, Thomas, and David Strömberg. 2007. "News Droughts, News Floods, and US Disaster Relief." *Quarterly Journal of Economics* 122, no. 2: 693–728.

Enns, Peter K. 2014. "The Public's Increasing Punitiveness and Its Influence on Mass Incarceration in the United States." *American Journal of Political Science* 58, no. 4: 857–72.

Enns, Peter K. 2016. *Incarceration Nation.* Cambridge: Cambridge University Press.

FDA (Federal Drug Administration). 2019. "Timeline of Selected FDA Activities and Significant Events Addressing Opioid Misuse and Abuse." www.fda.gov /downloads/Drugs/DrugSafety/InformationbyDrugClass/UCM566985.pdf (accessed April 11, 2019).

Fellowes, Matthew C., and Gretchen Rowe. 2004. "Politics and the New American Welfare States." *American Journal of Political Science* 48, no. 2: 362–73.

Fowler, Anthony, and Andrew B. Hall. 2016. "The Elusive Quest for Convergence." *Quarterly Journal of Political Science* 11, no. 1: 131–49.

Frost, Karen, Erica Frank, and Edward Maibach. 1997. "Relative Risk in the News Media: A Quantification of Misrepresentation." *American Journal of Public Health* 87, no. 5: 842–45.

Fryer, Roland G., Paul S. Heaton, Steven D. Levitt, and Kevin M. Murphy. 2013. "Measuring Crack Cocaine and Its Impact." *Economic Inquiry* 51, no. 3: 1651–81.

Gallup. 2019. "Most Important Problem." news.gallup.com/poll/1675/most-important -problem.aspx (accessed January 11, 2019).

Gentzkow, Matthew, and Jesse M. Shapiro. 2008. "Introduction of Television to the United States Media Market, 1946–1960." Ann Arbor, MI: Inter-university Consortium for Political and Social Research (distributor), September 30. doi.org/ 10.3886/ICPSR22720.v1.

Gilens, Martin, and Benjamin I. Page. 2014. "Testing Theories of American Politics: Elites, Interest Groups, and Average Citizens." *Perspectives on Politics* 12, no. 3: 564–81.

Gilliam Jr., Franklin D., and Shanto Iyengar. 2000. "Prime Suspects: The Influence of Local Television News on the Viewing Public." *American Journal of Political Science* 44, no. 3: 560–73.

Glanton, Dahleen. 2017. "Race, the Crack Epidemic, and the Effect on Today's Opioid Crisis." *Chicago Tribune*, August 21. www.chicagotribune.com/columns/dahleen -glanton/ct-opioid-epidemic-dahleen-glanton-met-20170815-column.html.

Golub, Andrew Lang, and Bruce D. Johnson. 1997. "Crack's Decline: Some Surprises across US Cities." National Institute of Justice, July. www.ncjrs.gov/pdffiles /165707.pdf.

Grose, Christian R., and Bruce I. Oppenheimer. 2007. "The Iraq War, Partisanship, and Candidate Attributes: Variation in Partisan Swing in the 2006 US House Elections." *Legislative Studies Quarterly* 32, no. 4: 531–57.

Harbin, M. Brielle. 2018. "The Contingency of Compassion in Media Depictions of Drug Addiction." Paper presented at the American Political Science Association Political Communications Pre-Conference Meeting, Harvard University, Cambridge, MA, August 29.

Hartman, Donna M., and Andrew Golub. 1999. "The Social Construction of the Crack Epidemic in the Print Media." *Journal of Psychoactive Drugs* 31, no. 4: 423–33.

Hertel-Fernandez, Alexander, Matto Mildenberger, and Leah C. Stokes. 2019. "Legislative Staff and Representation in Congress." *American Political Science Review* 113, no. 1: 1–18.

Hurwitz, Jon, and Mark Peffley. 1997. "Public Perceptions of Race and Crime: The Role of Racial Stereotypes." *American Journal of Political Science* 41, no. 2: 375–401.

Katz, Josh, and Margot Sanger-Katz. 2018. "'The Numbers Are So Staggering.' Overdose Deaths Set a Record Last Year." *New York Times*, November 29. www .nytimes.com/interactive/2018/11/29/upshot/fentanyl-drug-overdose-deaths.html.

Keller, Jared. 2017. "A Tale of Two Drug Wars." *Pacific Standard*, December 8. psmag .com/social-justice/a-tale-of-two-drug-wars.

King, Jamilah. 2017. "Senator Kamala Harris Blasts Racialized Double Standard of Crack and Opioid Epidemics." *Mic*, May 17. www.mic.com/articles/177298 /senator-kamala-harris-blasts-racialized-double-standard-of-crack-and-opioid -epidemics.

Kingdon, John W. 1984. *Agendas, Alternatives, and Public Policies*. Boston: Little, Brown.

Koger, Gregory. 2003. "Position Taking and Cosponsorship in the US House." *Legislative Studies Quarterly* 28, no. 2: 225–46.

Kolhatkar, Sheelah. 2017. "The Cost of the Opioid Crisis." *New Yorker*, September 18. www.newyorker.com/magazine/2017/09/18/the-cost-of-the-opioid-crisis.

Kriner, Douglas, and Francis Shen. 2014. "Responding to War on Capitol Hill: Battlefield Casualties, Congressional Response, and Public Support for the War in Iraq." *American Journal of Political Science* 58, no. 1: 157–74.

Lazarus, Jeffrey. 2013. "Issue Salience and Bill Introduction in the House and Senate." *Congress and the Presidency* 40, no. 3: 215–29.

Lopez, German. 2017. "When a Drug Epidemic's Victims Are White." Vox.com, April 4. www.vox.com/identities/2017/4/4/15098746/opioid-heroin-epidemic-race.

Mauer, Marc, and Tracy Huling. 1995. "Young Black Americans and the Criminal Justice System: Five Years Later." Sentencing Project, October. www.sentencing project.org/wp-content/uploads/2016/01/Young-Black-Americans-and-the-Criminal -Justice-System-Five-Years-Later.pdf.

McKenzie, Kevin. 2017. "Largely White Opioid Epidemic Highlights Black Frustration with Drug War." *Commercial Appeal*, March 26. www.commercialappeal .com/story/money/2017/03/26/white-opioid-epidemic-highlights-black-frustration -drug-war/97694296/.

Miler, Kristina C. 2018. *Poor Representation: Congress and the Politics of Poverty in the United States.* Cambridge: Cambridge University Press.

Mummolo, Jonathan, and Erik Peterson. 2018. "Improving the Interpretation of Fixed Effects Regression Results." *Political Science Research and Methods* 6, no. 4: 829–35.

Murakawa, Naomi. 2011. "Toothless: The Methamphetamine 'Epidemic,' 'Meth Mouth,' and the Racial Construction of Drug Scares." *Du Bois Review: Social Science Research on Race* 8, no. 1: 219–28.

NCSL (National Council of State Legislatures). 2017. "Prescribing Policies: States Confront Opioid Overdose Epidemic." June 30. www.ncsl.org/research/health /prescribing-policies-states-confront-opioid-overdose-epidemic.aspx.

Netherland, Julie, and Helena B. Hansen. 2016. "The War on Drugs That Wasn't: Wasted Whiteness, 'Dirty Doctors,' and Race in Media Coverage of Prescription Opioid Misuse." *Culture, Medicine, and Psychiatry* 40, no. 4: 664–86.

Newkirk, Vann R. 2017. "What the 'Crack Baby' Panic Reveals about the Opioid Epidemic." *Atlantic*, July 16. www.theatlantic.com/politics/archive/2017/07/what -the-crack-baby-panic-reveals-about-the-opioid-epidemic/533763/.

Overby, L. Marvin, and Kenneth M. Cosgrove. 1996. "Unintended Consequences? Racial Redistricting and the Representation of Minority Interests." *Journal of Politics* 58, no. 2: 540–50.

Parker, Andrew M., Daniel Strunk, and David A. Fiellin. 2018. "State Responses to the Opioid Crisis." *Journal of Law, Medicine, and Ethics* 46, no. 2: 367–81.

Peltzman, Sam. 1984. "Constituent Interest and Congressional Voting." *Journal of Law and Economics* 27, no. 1: 181–210.

Peterson, Kristina, and Stephanie Armour. 2018. "Opioid vs. Crack: Congress Reconsiders Its Approach to Drug Epidemic." *Wall Street Journal*, May 5.

Pew Research Center. 2014. "America's Changing Drug Policy Landscape: Two-Thirds Favor Treatment, Not Jail, for Use of Heroin, Cocaine." US Politics and Policy, April 2. www.people-press.org/2014/04/02/americas-new-drug-policy -landscape/.

Poole, Keith T., and Howard Rosenthal. 2007. *Ideology and Congress.* New Brunswick, NJ: Transaction Publishers.

Rothwell, Jonathan. 2015. "Drug Offenders in American Prisons: The Critical Distinction between Stock and Flow." Brookings Institution, November 25. archive .today/hWMQY.

Scholl, Lawrence, Puja Seth, Mbabazi Kariisa, Nana Otoo Wilson, and Grant Baldwin. 2018. "Drug and Opioid-Involved Overdose Deaths—United States, 2013–2017." *Morbidity and Mortality Weekly Report* 67, nos. 51–52: 1419–27.

Shihipar, Abdullah. 2019. "The Opioid Crisis Isn't White." *New York Times*, February 26.

Snyder, James M., and David Strömberg. 2010. "Press Coverage and Political Accountability." *Journal of Political Economy* 118, no. 2: 355–408.

Stewart, Charles, and Jonathan Woon. n.d. "Congressional Committee Assignments, 103rd to 115th Congresses, 1993–2017." Electronic data, 103rd–115th Congresses. web.mit.edu/17.251/www/data_page.html (accessed January 14, 2020).

Swift, Elaine K., Robert G. Brookshire, David T. Canon, Evelyn C. Fink, John R. Hibbing, Brian D. Humes, Michael J. Malbin, and Kenneth C. Martis. 2000. "Database of Congressional Historical Statistics." Computer file. Ann Arbor, MI: Inter-university Consortium for Political and Social Research (distributor).

Volden, Craig, and Alan E. Wiseman. 2014. *Legislative Effectiveness in the United States Congress: The Lawmakers.* Cambridge: Cambridge University Press.

Waggoner, Philip D. 2019. "Do Constituents Influence Issue-Specific Bill Sponsorship?" *American Politics Research* 47, no. 4: 709–38.

Weaver, David, Maxwell McCombs, and Donald L. Shaw. 2004. "Agenda-Setting Research: Issues, Attributes, and Influences." In *Handbook of Political Communication Research*, edited by Lynda Lee Kaid, chapter 10 (ebook). New York: Routledge.

Winburn, Jonathan, and Jas M. Sullivan. 2011. "The Significance of Race and Geography on Legislative Behavior: Exploring the Legislative Agenda in Post-Katrina Louisiana." *Journal of Black Studies* 42, no. 5: 791–810.

Xie, Tao. 2006. "Congressional Roll Call Voting on China Trade Policy." *American Politics Research* 34, no. 6: 732–58.

Criminal Justice or Public Health: A Comparison of the Representation of the Crack Cocaine and Opioid Epidemics in the Media

Carmel Shachar
Harvard University

Tess Wise
Amherst College

Gali Katznelson
Western University

Andrea Louise Campbell
Massachusetts Institute of Technology

Abstract

Context: The opioid epidemic is a major US public health crisis. Its scope prompted significant public outreach, but this response triggered a series of journalistic articles comparing the opioid epidemic to the crack cocaine epidemic. Some authors claimed that the political response to the crack cocaine epidemic was criminal justice rather than medical in nature, motivated by divergent racial demographics.

Methods: We examine these assertions by analyzing the language used in relevant newspaper articles. Using a national sample, we compare word frequencies from articles about crack cocaine in 1988–89 and opioids in 2016–17 to evaluate media framings. We also examine articles about methamphetamines in 1992–93 and heroin throughout the three eras to distinguish between narratives used to describe the crack cocaine and opioid epidemics.

Findings: We find support for critics' hypotheses about the differential framing of the two epidemics: articles on the opioid epidemic are likelier to use medical terminology than criminal justice terminology while the reverse is true for crack cocaine articles.

Conclusions: Our analysis suggests that race and legality may influence policy responses to substance-use epidemics. Comparisons also suggest that the evolution of the media narrative on substance use cannot alone account for the divergence in framing between the two epidemics.

Keywords media narratives, public health model of substance use, criminal justice model of substance use, crack cocaine epidemic, opioid epidemic

Journal of Health Politics, Policy and Law, Vol. 45, No. 2, April 2020
DOI 10.1215/03616878-8004862   © 2020 by Duke University Press

The opioid epidemic is one of the most significant public health crises in the United States today. Of the more than 70,200 drug overdose deaths in 2017, around 68% were attributed to opioid abuse (CDC 2018). The statistical trends regarding the epidemic are equally alarming; in 2017, the number of overdose deaths involving opioids was six times higher than in 1999 (CDC 2018). The worrying scope of the epidemic has prompted significant public outreach, including the White House declaring the epidemic a public health emergency while calling for better controls of prescription medications and access to substance-use treatment facilities (Davis 2017). Congress likewise allocated funding to treat the opioid epidemic as a public health concern and not a criminal justice issue in the 21st Century Cures Act, enacted in December 2016. State governments have also responded to the opioid epidemic through public health initiatives. For example, in 2017 Illinois released an Opioid Action Plan not through its law enforcement agencies but through its Department of Public Health, noting "The focus of our efforts is to save lives" (Rauner 2017). The messaging is clear: substance use is a medical, not a law enforcement, issue.

The rise in public health–focused responses to the opioid epidemic triggered a series of journalistic articles and opinion pieces comparing the epidemic to the earlier crack cocaine epidemic. Titles of these pieces included "America's Racist Response to the Crack Epidemic Must Inform the Way We Tackle Opioids" (Sharpton 2018) and "Why Didn't My Drug-Affected Family Get Any Sympathy?" (Bailey 2018). The authors of these pieces compared the criminal justice response to the crack cocaine epidemic of the 1980s with the public health approach to the current opioid epidemic and concluded that the differences in framing and public policy solutions were motivated by racism. Specifically, they were concerned that the differential responses were due to an association between crack cocaine and African Americans while the opioid epidemic is now seen as a problem afflicting white communities.

This article examines these assertions by analyzing the language used in newspaper articles from each period. Drawing on newspapers across the country, we compare word frequencies from articles about crack cocaine in 1988–89 and opioids in 2016–17 to evaluate how each epidemic was framed in public discourse. We particularly examine language indicating a medical model of addiction, such as health and treatment, as compared to terms of social control, such as police, enforcement, and arrest. We find support for the critics' hypothesis about the differential framing of the two substance-use epidemics: articles on the opioid epidemic are more likely to use medical or public health terminology—and evince concern about people. By contrast, articles on the crack cocaine epidemic utilize criminal justice terms and evoke concerns about drugs more frequently. To better understand the role that type of substance and race of users associated with the epidemic plays, we also examined articles about the methamphetamine epidemic from 1992–93, as this is an epidemic that has been associated with white users (as with opioids) but focuses on a stimulant (similar to crack cocaine). To better trace shifts in narratives, we pulled articles focusing specifically on heroin use from 1988–89, 1992–93, and 2016–17. The framing of the two epidemics, especially in contrast to articles written during these two periods about heroin, suggests that the evolution of understanding substance use disorders is not the sole explanation for the difference in media narratives. Instead, another factor, such as street drug status or race, may play a role in the public policy response and outreach to substance-use epidemics.

Public Policy, Substance Use, and Media Narratives

The media influences public policy agendas by prioritizing some news topics over others and therefore influencing which issues the public consider important (McCombs 1993). The media also has the ability to frame issues by influencing the perceptions the public and key policy makers have on topics as well as suggesting appropriate responses and solutions (Bennett 1990, 2016; Busby, Flynn, and Druckman 2018; Scheufele and Tewksbury 2007). This influence may be particularly strong on complicated public policy issues, such as poverty and welfare programs. For example, there is evidence that media framing connecting social welfare programs to race can shift public opinion and, in turn, public policies on the best way to address poverty alleviation (Winter 2006).

The media's effectiveness in setting agendas and framing issues is well documented in public responses to health issues (Brodie 2003). The ability of mass media to influence the perceptions regarding substance users and drive policy is no exception. As early as 1963, Howard Becker illustrated the role that media played in shaping the perception of drug users—in his case marijuana users—as deviant (Becker 1963). Criminal justice historians have documented that politicians and media often construct a narrative of drug use that presents substance use as a criminal act rather than one that arises from a medical disorder. Although the "just say no" era of the 1980s and 1990s is the most popular example of the criminalization model of substance use, it is prevalent throughout US political history. For example, the enactment of harsh mandatory minimum sentencing laws for marijuana and heroin occurred in the 1950s, when the dominant narrative around substance use was that foreign pushers were inflicting substances on defenseless Americans (Lassiter 2015).

The model used to frame a substance use epidemic is crucial because it not only shapes public perception of the epidemic but also public policy responses. By linking substance use and crime, the criminalization model drives draconian and drastic solutions to the use of illicit substances. Examples of these public policy interventions include mandatory sentencing, "three strikes and you're out" policies, and even the use of the death penalty in some substance use cases (Krisberg 2015). These policies are often promoted under a "get tough on crime" campaign that can also drive the rise of a police state, with more funding to law enforcement, more criminal prosecutions, and higher rates of incarceration (Messner and Rosenfeld 2007). Unfortunately, the public policy interventions often justified by the criminalization model have been shown to have little impact on rates of serious crime (Messner and Rosenfeld 2007). They do come with important concerns regarding civil rights and liberties, however. For example, likely due to rhetoric based in the criminalization model of substance use in the 1980s, the percentage of Americans who felt that testing workers for substance use in general would be an unfair invasion of privacy declined from 44 percent in 1986 to 24 percent in 1989 (Beckett 1994).

The medical model of substance use disorder calls for very different interventions. Instead of adopting a "tough on crime" stance, policy makers influenced by the medicalization model respond with offers of help, including resources for treatment and prevention (Netherland and Hansen 2017). Treatment interventions include diverting substance users from prisons to rehabilitation facilities, sometimes through drug courts. Prevention policies include prescription drug monitoring programs to limit the number of opioid prescriptions in a community as well as educational efforts around substance use. There is an understanding under this model that substance users are victims of their own biology. Blame may be shifted from the user to the supplier—either the pharmaceutical industry, physicians who are careless with their prescriptions, or illicit drug sellers (Macy 2018). A telling outgrowth of the focus on the supply side of substance use is the rise of prescription drug monitoring programs, funded by the 2005 National All Schedules Prescription Reporting Act and present in 49 states (Oliva 2018). These programs are intended to reduce the availability of opioids by requiring prescribers to report the number of opioid prescriptions they write for patients, suggesting a perception that overeager providers—and not users seeking out opioids—are the driver of opioid use. Overall, the medicalization model is kinder to substance users in that it encourages policy makers to provide health care resources to support recovery rather than harsher criminal justice interventions.

Race, Substance Use, and Media Narratives

Layered on top of media narratives and frames around substance use in the United States is the role of race. Evidence suggests that the nature of racial content influences which media framing resonates most strongly with the public and becomes the dominant narrative. While some of this response may be motivated by explicitly racist biases, most is likely a result of implicit (Beckett, Nyrop, and Pfingst 2006: 106) and structural biases (Bobo and Thompson 2006). Racial cues can feed into the perception of the severity of a crime or social problem (Beckett, Nyrop, and Pfingst 2006: 107). In the case of substance use, associating addiction with communities of color can persuade the public and policy makers that substance use causes violence, crime, and other problematic behaviors. An association between race and addiction can give media narratives that emphasize the criminalization model of substance use greater resonance among policy makers and the public alike.

Indeed, Michelle Alexander (2012) argues that today's mass incarceration of African Americans originates in a deliberate strategy of the Reagan administration to link substance use, criminality, and race in media narratives in order to drum up public and congressional support for the War on Drugs, announced in 1982. Capitalizing on backlash against the civil rights movement of the 1960s, conservative politicians beginning with Richard Nixon and his Southern Strategy realized the political utility of using racial appeals to attract white voters (see also Mendelberg 2001). When it came into power, the Reagan administration deliberately sought to shape perceptions of drug users and views on drug policy, announcing the War on Drugs at a time when illegal drug use was actually declining (Alexander 2012: 6). The announcement predated the crack epidemic, but provided the pretext for mass imprisonment once crack began to spread in poor black neighborhoods.

The impact of the criminalization model of substance use on the African American community is significant. African Americans are incarcerated at more than five times the rate of whites (NAACP n.d.). While African Americans and whites use illicit drugs at similar rates, imprisonment rates for drug-related offenses are almost six times higher for African Americans than for whites, and while African Americans represent only 12.4% of illicit substance users, they constitute 33% of those incarcerated in state facilities for drug-related offenses (NAACP n.d.). The mass incarceration of African Americans for drug-related offenses also has serious collateral consequences, including exclusion from social supports such as financial aid and housing benefits, and challenges in achieving employment and financial security (National Research Council 2014), what Alexander terms "a new racial caste system" (2012: 3).

Even when white users fall under the criminalization model, they are often protected by their racial privilege. For example, when there was an outbreak of heroin use among white high school and college students in the Dallas area in the 1990s, the law enforcement response was to prosecute the Mexican cartels "preying on this community" (Lassiter 2015: 126). As a result, although whites represent a sizable majority of substance users and drug dealers in the United States, they compose only one-quarter of drug offenders in state prisons (127). Similarly, methamphetamine has been linked to white users, and therefore its users are often portrayed as deserving more sympathy, and less linked to violence than crack cocaine users are (Murakawa 2011). An analysis of media depictions of drug use during the first decade of the 2000s found that prescription opioid users were typically portrayed as white, suburban or rural, and deserving sympathy, while heroin users were usually described as black or Latino, urban, and criminal (Netherland and Hansen 2016).

Methods

To assess the extant hypothesis that the opioid and crack cocaine epidemics were differentially framed in the media, we drew articles from major US newspapers, including the *Chicago Tribune*, *Los Angeles Times*, *Newsday*, *St. Louis Post-Dispatch*, *Boston Globe*, *New York Times*, *Wall Street Journal*, and *Washington Post*. We had originally intended to use several regional newspapers, including from areas with high crack cocaine or opioid use, but were limited to the set of papers whose digital archives extended back sufficiently.

We narrowed our searches to two time periods, 1988–89 and 2016–17, to maximize similarities between the two epidemics. In 1988, during George H. W. Bush's election year, there was a surge in reporting on crack cocaine that continued into the first year of his administration (Reinarman and Levine 1997: 21). Because the 2016 election of another Republican candidate, Donald Trump, coincided with media attention to the opioid epidemic, we chose the years 2016–17 for comparison. To search for articles we used the search engine Lexis Advance. One search was for articles that included crack cocaine and that were published between January 1, 1988, and December 31, 1989. This search resulted in 2,055 articles from the selected newspapers. The other search was for articles that included opioid and that were published between January 1, 2016, and December 31, 2017. This search resulted in 4,026 articles.

We also pulled articles focusing on methamphetamines and heroin, to better capture a variety of factors and to serve as comparisons to the crack cocaine and opioid epidemics. Methamphetamine was selected as a drug epidemic that focused on a stimulant—similar in that respect to crack cocaine—but also as an epidemic that has often been associated primarily with white users (Murakawa 2011)—akin to the opioid epidemic. To search for articles on methamphetamine, we focused on 1992–93, because those years encompassed a presidential election and the start of a new administration under President William J. Clinton. We separated heroin from our opioid search, even though heroin is an opioid, in order to track the trajectory of a longer running epidemic as well as to compare the narratives around a street drug to a broader category of substances that include prescription medications.[1] Our searches for articles that focused on heroin use encompassed 1988–89, in order to serve as a temporal comparison to our crack cocaine search, 1992–93, to serve as a comparison to our methamphetamines search, and 2016–17, to serve as a comparison to our broader opioid search. There were 391 articles for the methamphetamine sample, 3,956 articles for heroin 1988–89, 2,865 for heroin 1992–93, and 4,112 articles for heroin 2016–17.

We compared the word frequencies in our samples using a variety of methods, including looking at relative word frequency and creating a topic model using Latent Dirichlet Allocation (LDA). LDA (Blei, Ng, and Jordan 2003; Pritchard et al. 2000) is a generative statistical model that posits that each document (newspaper article in our case) is a mixture of a number of topics and that each word in the document can be attributed to a particular topic. When using LDA, the distribution of topics is generally assumed to have a sparse Dirichlet prior, reflecting an assumption that documents cover only a small set of topics and that topics use only a small set of words frequently. In our case, such an assumption is reasonable because newspaper articles are generally narrowly focused and use common language. In LDA, topics are not semantically strongly defined and words may co-occur across different topics. A topic model allows us to see how topics vary across the 1988–89, 1992–92, and 2016–17 samples. Before

---

1. One might worry that separating heroin from opioids would bias the results in favor of a medical frame. At the suggestion of a helpful anonymous reviewer, we conducted an analysis of the combined sample of opioid and heroin articles for 2016–17. While the language in this combined sample does shift slightly toward a law enforcement frame, the medical theme continues to dominate as can be seen from the results in appendix A.

running the model, the samples were cleaned as follows: stopwords (and, the, it, etc.),[2] punctuation, and numbers were removed, and all words were converted to lowercase.[3]

Findings

The most frequently occurring words in the 1988–89 crack cocaine sample (see table 1) included language relating to criminal justice such as police, law, enforcement, and crime. The emphasis on criminal justice continued through our bigram analysis of the 1988–89 crack cocaine sample, with law + enforcement, substances + crime, drug + trafficking, drug + dealers, and illegal + drugs constituting half of the top ten. The trend continued in the trigram analysis of this sample, with controlled + substances + crime, special + investigative + forces, law + enforcement + officials, and law + court + tribunals.

By contrast, the most frequently occurring word in the 2016–17 opioids sample (see table 2) was health. Our bigram analysis of this sample also emphasized the rise of medical terminology, with health + care, public + health, and health + departments included in the top ten. The trigram analysis was the most heavily weighted toward medical language, with affordable + care + act, health + care + reform, public + health + administration, health + care + policy, substance + abuse + treatment, and health + care + law comprising the majority of the top ten. Criminal justice terms did linger somewhat, including abuse, law + enforcement, and controlled + substances + crime, but were much less prevalent in the 2016–17 opioid sample than in the earlier crack cocaine sample.

Although the unigram analysis of the 1992–93 methamphetamine sample (table 3) only includes two criminal justice words (police and court), the bigram analysis is largely dominated by criminal justice phrases, including law + enforcement, and pleaded + guilty. The trigram analysis consists entirely of criminal justice phrases, both ones that appear in the 1988–89 crack cocaine sample (law + enforcement + officials) and ones that are unique to this sample (fourth + reich + skinheads). Nevertheless, some key criminal justice words and phrases that dominate the crack cocaine

2. We developed a custom list of stopwords that included words associated with newspaper formatting (e.g., section, byline, graphic) in addition to three common libraries of stopwords (onix, SMART, and snowball) found in the R package "stopwords" (Benoit, Muhr, and Watanabe 2017).

3. We chose not to "stem" or "lemmatize" the words (e.g., substance and substances could be reduced to *substanc*) for ease of interpretation and integrity to the original texts, especially for bigrams and trigrams.

Table 1   Top Words in the 1988–89 Crack Cocaine Sample
(Unigram, Bigram, and Trigram)

Rank	Word	Frequency
1	drug	4650
2	cocaine	2584
3	police	2226
4	drugs	1924
5	crack	1764
6	people	1388
7	abuse	892
8	law	889
9	enforcement	841
10	crime	828

Rank	Word	Word	Frequency
1	law	enforcement	468
2	substance	abuse	406
3	substances	crime	369
4	controlled	substances	352
5	crack	cocaine	349
6	drug	trafficking	306
7	drug	dealers	263
8	drug	abuse	248
9	illegal	drugs	200
10	drug	policy	171

Rank	Word	Word	Word	Frequency
1	controlled	substances	crime	343
2	drug	enforcement	administration	113
3	special	investigative	forces	83
4	law	enforcement	officials	69
5	law	courts	tribunals	54
6	substance	abuse	treatment	43
7	students	student	life	39
8	national	football	league	38
9	substance	abuse	facilities	38
10	regional	local	governments	33

Note: Language related to criminal justice flagged in dark gray.

Table 2 Top Words in the 2016–17 Opioid Sample (Unigram, Bigram, and Trigram)

Rank	Word	Frequency
1	health	10652
2	drug	8987
3	opioid	6955
4	people	6045
5	care	5817
6	trump	4580
7	drugs	4364
8	public	3975
9	law	3713
10	abuse	3625

Rank	Word	Word	Frequency
1	health	care	3444
2	substance	abuse	1846
3	public	health	1832
4	opioid	crisis	1227
5	law	enforcement	1143
6	presidential	candidates	1066
7	health	departments	945
8	opioid	epidemic	883
9	white	house	836
10	donald	trump	753

Rank	Word	Word	Word	Frequency
1	affordable	care	act	560
2	health	care	reform	454
3	public	health	administration	443
4	controlled	substances	crime	442
5	health	care	policy	365
6	health	care	professionals	359
7	substance	abuse	treatment	352
8	health	care	law	334
9	special	investigative	forces	246
10	drug	enforcement	administration	237

Note: Language related to health and medicine flagged in light gray.

word frequency analysis, such as crime, substance crime, drug trafficking, drug dealers, and illegal drugs, are missing from the methamphetamine word frequency analysis. There was an absence of public health or medical terms in all three analyses used for the methamphetamine sample.

The evolution of language in the samples of heroin articles from 1988–89, 1992–93, and 2016–17 shows elements observed in both the opioid sample and the crack cocaine sample. The unigram analyses of these three time periods (see table 4) include two criminal justice terms in 1988–89, only one criminal justice term in the next two periods, and no public health or medical terms. This stands in contrast to the 2016–17 opioid sample, which included four public health terms and no criminal justice terms (see table 2). The bigram analysis of the 1988–89 heroin sample (see table 5) does include one public health term (drug + treatment) but five criminal justice terms, similar to the 1988–89 crack cocaine bigram analysis (see table 1), which includes five criminal justice terms although no public health language. The 1992–93 and 2016–17 bigram analyses (see table 5) are closer to balanced, with three criminal justice terms and two public health terms. Interestingly, the 1988–89 heroin trigram analysis (see table 6) includes two public health terms, although the majority of the other top ten terms are criminal justice terms, whereas the 1992–93 trigram analysis includes no public health terms and is weighed heavily to criminal justice terms. The 2016–17 trigram analysis breaks down along similar lines to the 1988–89 trigram analysis for heroin. This is in sharp contrast to the trigram analysis of the 2016–17 opioid sample (see table 2), which is majority public health terms.

By comparing the relative frequencies of words in these samples, we can more clearly observe similarities and differences in the media narratives around these substance use epidemics. In the following figures, words that occur with similar frequency in both samples appear closer to the 45-degree line. Words that are more prominent in the first named sample occur above the line, and words that are more prominent in the second named sample occur below the line. High-frequency words in figures 1–3 almost uniformly suggest a criminalization model while high-frequency words more prominent in the opioids sample (below the 45-degree line) suggest a medicalization model.

In the unigram analysis (fig. 1), high frequency words drawn from articles written about the opioid epidemic include arrested and police, while words drawn from articles about crack cocaine include health, care, addiction, medicaid, and fentanyl. The criminalization model is further seen in the bigram analysis (fig. 2), with words such as law enforcement

Table 3   Top Words in the 1992–93 Methamphetamine Sample (Unigram, Bigram, and Trigram)

Rank	Word	Frequency
1	drug	838
2	nov	686
3	oct	677
4	police	624
5	methamphetamine	554
6	sep	397
7	court	393
8	drugs	368
9	people	365
10	time	352

Rank	Word	Word	Frequency
1	child	abuse	69
2	law	enforcement	69
3	superior	court	62
4	antelope	valley	58
5	pleaded	guilty	57
6	dist	atty	52
7	sheriff's	department	49
8	court	judge	46
9	santa	ana	46
10	task	force	45

Rank	Word	Word	Word	Frequency
1	deputy	dist	atty	39
2	superior	court	judge	33
3	district	attorney's	office	22
4	drug	enforcement	administration	22
5	law	enforcement	officials	19
6	fourth	reich	skinheads	15
7	chula	vista	police	14
8	u.s	district	court	13
9	u.s	attorney's	office	12
10	handler	unknown	materials	11

Note: Language related to criminal justice flagged in dark gray.

Table 4 Top Words in the 1988–89, 1992–93, and 2016–17 Heroin Samples (Unigrams)

1988–89

Rank	Word	Frequency
1	drug	22523
2	drugs	9767
3	heroin	8417
4	police	8169
5	people	7798
6	cocaine	7504
7	time	5425
8	crack	4306
9	document	4063
10	federal	4062

1992–93

Rank	Word	Frequency
1	drug	11017
2	heroin	5860
3	people	5749
4	police	5634
5	drugs	4626
6	time	4214
7	life	3275
8	document	2931
9	cocaine	2719
10	home	2595

2016–17

Rank	Word	Frequency
1	drug	13688
2	people	10833
3	police	10264
4	heroin	10111
5	drugs	6159
6	opioid	5995
7	time	5846
8	addiction	5108
9	health	4776
10	treatment	4622

Note: Language related to criminal justice flagged in dark gray.

Table 5 Top Words in the 1988–89, 1992–93, and 2016–17 Heroin Samples (Bigrams)

1988–89

Rank	Word	Word	Frequency
1	law	enforcement	1434
2	drug	abuse	1312
3	drug	dealers	953
4	drug	treatment	815
5	drug	enforcement	789
6	drug	users	671
7	drug	related	565
8	drug	trafficking	561
9	anti	drug	554
10	police	officers	491

1992–93

Rank	Word	Word	Frequency
1	law	enforcement	960
2	drug	abuse	451
3	drug	enforcement	446
4	drug	dealers	422
5	task	force	363
6	police	officers	344
7	series	occasional	330
8	drug	treatment	329
9	health	care	311
10	drug	users	294

2016–17

Rank	Word	Word	Frequency
1	law	enforcement	960
2	drug	abuse	451
3	drug	enforcement	446
4	drug	dealers	422
5	task	force	363
6	police	officers	344
7	series	occasional	330
8	drug	treatment	329
9	health	care	311
10	drug	users	294

Note: Language related to criminal justice flagged in dark gray; language related to health and medicine flagged in light gray.

Table 6   Top Words in the 1988–89, 1992–93, and 2016–17 Heroin Samples (Trigrams)

1988–89

Rank	Word	Word	Word	Frequency
1	drug	enforcement	administration	472
2	law	enforcement	officials	397
3	intravenous	drug	users	185
4	drug	treatment	programs	166
5	u.s	district	court	164
6	u.s	drug	enforcement	139
7	world	war	ii	132
8	law	enforcement	agencies	129
9	substance	abuse	services	118
10	federal	drug	enforcement	114

1992–93

Rank	Word	Word	Word	Frequency
1	drug	enforcement	administration	262
2	law	enforcement	officials	261
3	u.s	attorney's	office	119
4	u.s	district	judge	116
5	world	war	ii	116
6	assistant	u.s	attorney	89
7	district	attorney's	office	80
8	u.s	district	court	78
9	criminal	justice	system	73
10	farrar	straus	giroux	71

2016–17

Rank	Word	Word	Word	Frequency
1	drug	enforcement	administration	320
2	law	enforcement	officials	267
3	district	attorney's	office	184
4	criminal	justice	system	180
5	affordable	care	act	165
6	degree	criminal	possession	159
7	drug	overdose	deaths	146
8	anthony	lamar	smith	129
9	public	health	officials	126
10	law	enforcement	agencies	119

Note: Language related to criminal justice flagged in dark gray; language related to health and medicine flagged in light gray.

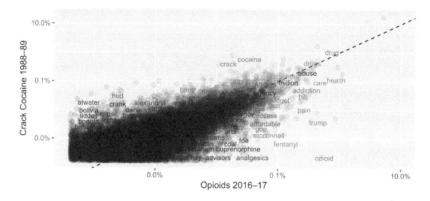

Figure 1 Relative frequencies of words in the 1988–89 crack cocaine and 2016–17 opioid samples (unigrams).

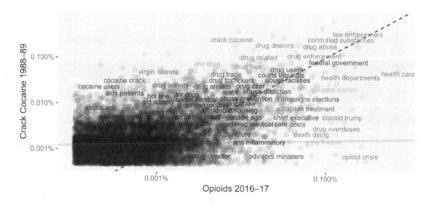

Figure 2 Relative frequencies of words in the 1988–89 crack cocaine and 2016–17 opioid samples (bigrams).

and drug trafficking from the crack cocaine articles, in comparison with the medicalized language of doctors and pain for the opioid sample. In the trigram analysis (fig. 3), expressions such as controlled substances crime stand out as associated with the crack cocaine epidemic as compared to health care professionals, which occurs with higher relative frequency in the opioids sample. Assertions that public discourse on the crack cocaine and opioid epidemics was different are upheld in this analysis of media coverage from each period.

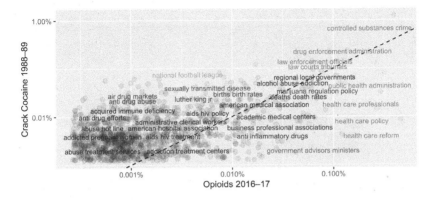

Figure 3   Relative frequencies of words in the 1988–89 crack cocaine and 2016–17 opioid samples (trigrams).

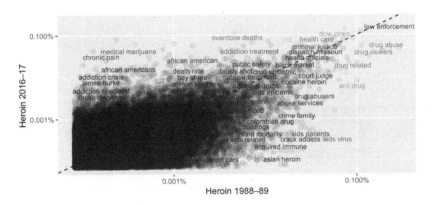

Figure 4   Relative frequencies of words in the 1988–89 and 2016–17 heroin samples (bigrams).

The trend away from criminal justice to public health and medical terms found in the relative frequencies comparisons between the crack cocaine and opioid samples was also found in the comparison of the relative frequencies of words in the 1988–89 and 2016–17 heroin samples (see fig. 4). Although these samples cover the same substance, the terminology used in 2016–17 was much more medical, such as addiction treatment, than the 1988–89 sample, which includes terms such as crime family and court judge. This suggests that the narrative around substance use overall was

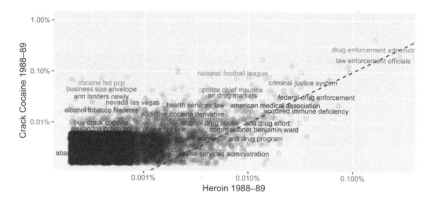

Figure 5 Relative frequencies of words in the 1988–89 crack cocaine and heroin samples (trigrams).

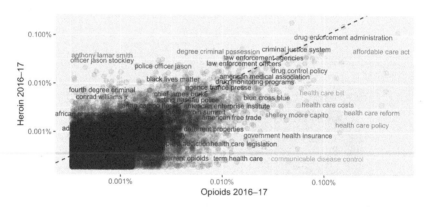

Figure 6 Relative frequencies of words in the 2016–17 heroin and opioid samples (trigrams).

shifting during this time period. This shift is also suggested by figure 5, which is the relative frequencies of words in the 1988–89 crack cocaine and 1988–89 heroin samples. In this figure, the words are clustered tightly around the dividing line, suggesting relatively little difference in the terminology used. The comparison between the 2016–17 heroin and opioid samples in figure 6 shows a little more divergence, on the other hand, with heroin being associated slightly more with criminal justice terminology and opioids being associated with health care terms.

Topic Models

Another way to see the divergence in rhetoric between the 1988–89 and 2016–17 samples is to use a topic model. As stated above, a topic model posits that each article is a mixture of a number of topics and that each word in the document can be attributed to one of the article's topics. Figures 7–10 show the results of topic models generated using LDA on the two samples. After repeated tests we chose to set the model to find three topics. This choice is justified by analyzing the Bayesian Information Criterion (BIC) associated with each model, which is an indicator of the trade-off between complexity and parsimony (Soleimani and Miller (2014). The BIC was minimized by either a two-topic model (for the crack cocaine 1988–89, opioids 2016–17, and methamphetamine 1992–93) or a three-topic model (for heroin 1988–89 and heroin 2019–17). To facilitate comparability, three-topic models were used for all, with the understanding that the third topic will vary in its coherence, often resembling a "remainder" category. The values in figures 7–10 are betas, which reflect the concentration of words in the topic.

In figure 7 (1988–89 crack cocaine sample) the three topics include two that are relatively coherent—topic 1 is a clear law-and-order topic with words such as law, enforcement, crime, and arrested. Topic 2 is centered around communities and families but includes the interesting additions of black and white, which are likely to touch on race. Topic 3 is less coherent, but seems to touch on government policy.

Figure 8, which shows the same analysis for the opioid sample (2016–17) has some overlap with the 1988–89 crack cocaine analysis in its topics— topic 1 is a community and home category (family, home, children) and topic 2 is still a political (trump, republican, government, policy) but topic 3 is clearly more medical than law enforcement (health, pain, addiction, patients, epidemic).[4] This analysis shows that when a three-topic model is considered the two samples differ strongly on topic 3 with the 1988–89 crack cocaine sample including a law enforcement topic and the 2016–17 opioid sample including a medical topic.

Performing the LDA topic model analysis for the 1992–93 methamphetamine sample (see figure 9) resulted in a very clear criminal justice topic (topic 3), a family and community topic that leaned in an interestingly

---

4. This is not to say that law enforcement is entirely absent, merely that it is a less prominent topic than health or politics. Adding a fourth topic to the model reveals a law enforcement–focused topic but with relatively low values of beta (i.e., words that occur less frequently) and at the expense of a higher (less desirable) BIC.

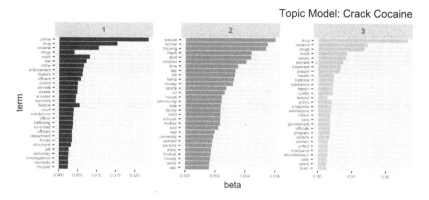

Figure 7 Topic model for the 1988–89 crack cocaine sample.

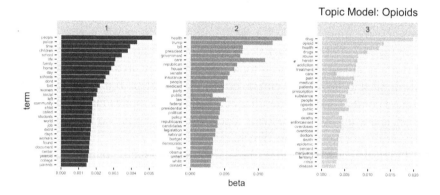

Figure 8 Topic model for the 2016–17 opioid sample.

negative direction, including words such as jail (topic 2), and a remainder topic that was relatively incoherent, as can be seen from the low values of beta (topic 1). Therefore, the topic model analysis for the methamphetamine sample was closer to the crack cocaine sample than to the opioid sample, despite the perception of both opioids and methamphetamine as white drugs. A key difference, however, between the topic model analyses for crack cocaine and for methamphetamine was that the criminal justice topic was topic 1 in the crack cocaine model but only topic 3 in the methamphetamine model, indicating that this topic was more prevalent in the framing of crack cocaine coverage.

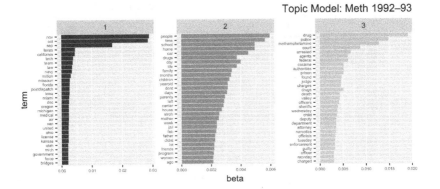

Figure 9   Topic model for the 1992–93 methamphetamine sample.

We performed the same analysis for the 1988–89 heroin sample and the 2016–17 heroin sample to compare them to the crack cocaine and opioid samples and also to compare them to each other to get a sense of any evolution in the media narrative between these two time periods. Figure 10 shows the analysis for the 1988–89 heroin sample. Topic 1 is very clearly a criminal justice topic with terms such as prison, crime, and criminal. Topic 2 again appears to be a community-focused topic, although, similar to the crack cocaine sample and not the opioid sample, it includes the term black, suggesting race. Topic 3 is focused around public health (with both public and health making an appearance) and treatment, which more closely aligns with the 2016–17 opioid analysis than the 1988–89 crack cocaine analysis. Figure 11 performs the sample analysis for the 2016–17 heroin sample. Topic 1 is a public health topic, while topic 3 appears to be a criminal justice topic. Topic 2 suggests a community and family focus with words such as school and mother and children.

The presence of both criminal justice and public health topics for both the 1988–89 and 2016–17 heroin samples is an interesting contrast to the topics for the crack cocaine and opioid samples.

With the heroin and crack cocaine samples, which both deal with illegal drugs purchased outside the medical system, we find criminal justice topics well represented. On the other hand, the opioid topic analysis does not yield a criminal justice topic. Using heroin in the two time periods as a control, we can see that the change from crack cocaine (with a criminal justice but no public health topic) to opioids (with no criminal justice but a public health topic) is not merely due to some secular change in increasing public health framings of drug epidemics. Heroin was around

Topic Model: Heroin 1988–89

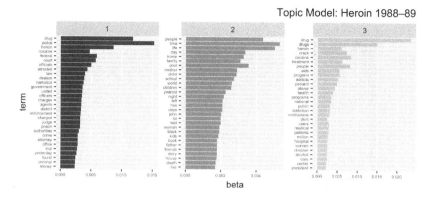

Figure 10   Topic model for the 1988–89 heroin sample.

Topic Model: Heroin 2016–17

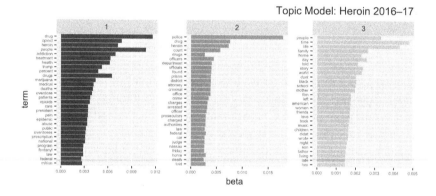

Figure 11   Topic model for the 2016–17 heroin sample.

in both eras, and had a public health framing in both eras. But opioids appear to be framed differently than crack, because crack had no public health framing back in 1988–89.

Conclusions

The word frequency patterns in the samples analyzed suggest a shift in the media narrative between the crack epidemic of the late 1980s to the more recent opioid epidemic. The 1988–89 crack cocaine sample demonstrates a strong criminalization focus, while the 2016–17 opioid sample illustrates the rise of the medicalization model. The analysis of the 1992–93 methamphetamine sample suggests that the criminalization narrative around substance use was still strong then. Tracing the narrative around heroin from 1988–89 through 1992–93 to 2016–17 provides an interesting contrast to the narratives utilized in the crack cocaine and opioid epidemics. The analysis of the 1988–89 heroin sample demonstrates that a public health framing was available during that time period and indeed appears in the topic models for 1988–89 heroin, but was not similarly used in the crack cocaine sample. While we observed both criminal justice and public health topics for heroin in both the earliest and latest heroin samples, we did not observe criminal justice or law enforcement topics appearing in the 2016–17 opioid sample. This suggests that the tone and content of media coverage of the opioid epidemic has indeed been different from both that of crack cocaine and that of heroin. Comparing the media narrative around heroin to the media narrative on the broader opioid epidemic in both 2016–17 samples indicates that the opioid epidemic has been consistently represented in more medicalized terms than other substance use epidemics.

While the framing around the epidemics has differed in public health versus law enforcement/criminal justice content, it is difficult to conclusively state whether the difference in narratives between the opioid epidemic and other substance use epidemics stems from the perception that the opioid epidemic is uniquely white. The heavy criminal justice narrative found in the 1992–93 methamphetamine sample, which was also a substance use epidemic associated with Caucasians, suggests otherwise. Furthermore, topic modeling indicates that criminal justice framing was more prevalent for the crack cocaine sample than for the methamphetamine sample, although it was present in both. Additionally, there is a distinction between opioid use and heroin use, which may reflect who we expect to be using each substance or our perception between users of prescription and illegal drugs. It could be that in order for the media narrative to shift, two factors were needed: an overall reframing of substance use as a public health issue that occurred at some point after 1992–93 and a perception that most users of the particular substance are white.

Interestingly, previous work analyzing the portrayal of the opioid epidemic may explain the shift in models between the opioid epidemic and other substance use epidemics. Emma McGinty et al. (2016) conducted an analysis of media coverage of opioid abuse from 1998 to 2012, focusing on whether law enforcement solutions (suggesting a criminalization model) or prevention-oriented solutions (suggesting a medicalization model) were proposed. Prior to 2007, news stories were much more likely to focus on law enforcement solutions to opioid use. The gap between the two types of solutions narrowed in 2007–09, and in 2010–12 the two types of solutions were represented with near equal frequency. We know that between 1993 and 2009 prescription opioid overdose admissions for whites increased 7.5 times, outstripping the rates of increase for African Americans (3.3) and Hispanics (3.2), and that since 2008, heroin-related overdose hospitalization rates for whites exceeded that of African Americans (Unick et al. 2013). While the shift in media narratives documented from 1998 to 2012 by McGinty et al. (2016) and then suggested for 2016–17 in the present article may be attributable to a variety of causes, it is likely that the changed demographics of addiction during this time period helped shift the trend away from law enforcement solutions to prevention-oriented solutions.

Media narratives matter because they shape and are bellwethers of solutions to public policy problems. A dominant narrative that substance use is a criminal justice issue is problematic because it can escalate law enforcement interventions that are ineffective and that raise serious civil rights concerns. Furthermore, a criminalization model of substance use reinforced by racial bias can contribute to the high rates of incarceration of people of color, especially African Americans. By contrast, a medicalization model of substance use promotes more effective public health interventions. In the samples we reviewed, the contrast of models was noticeable and lends credence to the popular hypothesis that the opioid epidemic is perceived and framed differently because of the demographic groups it impacts. This is especially notable when contrasted to previous works that documented a shift from criminalization to medicalization in the opioid epidemic media narratives at the same time that the rates of use among white Americans began to skyrocket. These findings, reinforcing the connection between race and public policy responses, may also have implications for other complex public policy issues that involve structural factors and are framed differently depending on the racial group most impacted, such as education policies including busing and welfare programs to address poverty.

■ ■ ■

Carmel Shachar is the executive director of the Petrie-Flom Center for Health Law Policy, Biotechnology, and Bioethics at Harvard Law School. Her research interests include the regulation of value-based health care, access to care for underserved populations, and the framing of a right to health care.
cshachar@law.harvard.edu

Tess Wise is a visiting professor of political science at Amherst College. Her research interests are US politics, the politics of consumer finance, race and US politics, political methodology, and political ethnography. She obtained her PhD from the Harvard University Department of Government in 2019.

Gali Katznelson is a medical student at the Schulich School of Medicine and Dentistry at Western University. She has a master's degree in bioethics from Harvard Medical School and was a student fellow at the Petrie-Flom Center for Health Law Policy, Biotechnology, and Bioethics at Harvard Law School.

Andrea Louise Campbell is Sloan Professor of Political Science at the Massachusetts Institute of Technology. Her interests include US politics, political behavior, public opinion, political inequality, and policy feedbacks. She is the author of *How Policies Make Citizens: Senior Citizen Activism and the American Welfare State* (2003), *The Delegated Welfare State: Medicare, Markets, and the Governance of Social Policy*, with Kimberly J. Morgan (2011), and *Trapped in America's Safety Net: One Family's Struggle* (2014). Funders include the National Science Foundation, the Robert Wood Johnson Foundation, and the Russell Sage Foundation. She is a member of the American Academy of Arts and Sciences.

Acknowledgments

We would like to thank the attendees of the Politics of the Opioid Epidemic conference, hosted at Brown University in collaboration with *JHPPL*, for their great feedback on our initial presentation of this work. Similarly, we would like to thank Eric Patashnik and Susan Moffitt for organizing the conference and for this opportunity. Lastly, we would like to thank our reviewer for his or her extremely helpful, thorough, and thoughtful comments.

References

Alexander, Michelle. 2012. *The New Jim Crow: Mass Incarceration in the Age of Colorblindness*. Rev. ed. New York: New Press.

Bailey, Issaac J. 2018. "Why Didn't My Drug-Affected Family Get Any Sympathy?" *Politico Magazine*, June 10. www.politico.com/magazine/story/2018/06/10/opioid -crisis-crack-crisis-race-donald-trump-218602.

Becker, Howard. 1963. *Outsiders: Studies in the Sociology of Deviance*. New York: Free Press.

Beckett, Katherine. 1994. "Setting the Public Agenda: 'Street Crime' and Drug Use in American Politics." *Social Problems* 41, no. 3: 425–47.

Beckett, Katherine, Kris Nyrop, and Lori Pfingst. 2006. "Race, Drugs, and Policing: Understanding Disparities in Drug Delivery Arrests." *Criminology* 44, no. 1: 105–37.

Bennett, W. Lance. 1990. "Toward a Theory of Press-State Relations in the United States." *Journal of Communication* 43, no. 4: 103–27.

Bennett, W. Lance. 2016. "Indexing Theory." In *The International Encyclopedia of Political Communication*, edited by Gianpietro Mazzoleni, Kevin G. Barnhurst, Ken'ichi Ikeda, Rousily C. M. Maia, and Hartmut Wesler, 513–17. New York: John Wiley and Sons.

Benoit, Kenneth, David Muhr, and Kohei Watanabe. 2017. "Stopwords: Multilingual Stopword Lists." R package version 0.9.0. CRAN.R-project.org/package=stopwords (accessed October 21, 2019).

Blei, David M., Andrew Y. Ng, and Michael I. Jordan. 2003. "Latent Dirichlet Allocation." *Journal of Machine Learning Research* 3: 993–1022.

Bobo, Lawrence D., and Victor Thompson. 2006. "Unfair by Design: The War on Drugs, Race, and the Legitimacy of the Criminal Justice System." *Social Research: An International Quarterly* 73, no. 2: 445–72.

Brodie, Mollyann, Elizabeth C. Hamel, and Drew E. Altman. 2003. "Health News and the American Public, 1996–2002." *Journal of Health Politics, Policy and Law* 28, no. 5: 927–50.

Busby, Ethan, D. J. Flynn, and James N. Druckman. 2018. "Studying Framing Effects on Political Preferences: Existing Research and Lingering Questions." In *Doing News Framing Analysis II*, edited by Paul D'Angelo, 27–50. New York: Routledge.

CDC (Centers for Disease Control and Prevention). 2018. "Understanding the Epidemic." www.cdc.gov/drugoverdose/epidemic/index.html (accessed January 14, 2019).

Davis, Julie Hirschfeld. 2017. "Trump Declares Opioid Crisis a 'Health Emergency' but Requests No Funds." *New York Times*, October 26. www.nytimes.com/2017/10 /26/us/politics/trump-opioid-crisis.html.

Krisberg, Barry A., Susan Marchionna, and Christopher Hartney. 2015. *American Corrections: Concepts and Controversies.* Thousand Oaks, CA: Sage Publications.

Lassiter, Matthew D. 2015. "Impossible Criminals: The Suburban Imperatives of America's War on Drugs." *Journal of American History* 102, no. 1: 126–40.

Macy, Beth. 2018. *Dopesick: Dealers, Doctors, and the Drug Company That Addicted America.* New York: Little, Brown and Company.

McCombs, Maxwell E., and Donald L. Shaw. 1993. "The Evolution of Agenda-Setting Research: Twenty-Five Years in the Marketplace of Ideas." *Journal of Communication* 43, no. 2: 58–67.

McGinty, Emma E., Alene Kennedy-Hendricks, Julia Baller, Jeff Niederdeppe, Sarah Gollust, and Colleen L. Barry. 2016. "Criminal Activity or Treatable Health Condition? New Media Framing of Opioid Analgesic Abuse in the United States, 1998–2012." *Psychiatric Services* 67, no. 4: 405–11.

Mendelberg, Tali. 2001. *The Race Card: Campaign Strategy, Implicit Messages, and the Norm of Equality.* Princeton, NJ: Princeton University Press.

Messner, Steve F., and Richard Rosenfeld. 2007. *Crime and the American Dream.* 4th ed. Belmont, CA: Wadsworth/Thomson Learning.

Murakawa, Naomi. 2011. "Toothless." *Du Bois Review: Social Science Research on Race* 8, no. 1: 219–28.

NAACP (National Association for the Advancement of Colored People). n.d. "Criminal Justice Fact Sheet." www.naacp.org/criminal-justice-fact-sheet/ (accessed January 23, 2019).

National Research Council. 2014. *The Growth of Incarceration in the United States: Exploring Causes and Consequences.* Washington, DC: National Academies Press.

Netherland, Julie, and Helena B. Hansen. 2016. "The War on Drugs That Wasn't: Wasted Whiteness, 'Dirty Doctors,' and Race in Media Coverage of Prescription Opioid Misuse." *Culture, Medicine, and Psychiatry* 40, no. 4: 664–86.

Netherland, Julie, and Helena B. Hansen. 2017. "White Opioids: Pharmaceutical Race and the War on Drugs That Wasn't." *BioSocieties* 12, no. 2: 217–38.

Oliva, Jennifer D. 2018. "Prescription Drug Policing: The Right to Protected Health Information Privacy Pre- and Post-Carpenter." *SSRN*, August 20. dx.doi.org/10.2139/ssrn.3225000.

Pritchard, Jonathan K., Matthew Stephens, Noah A. Rosenberg, and Peter Donnelly. 2000. "Association Mapping in Structured Populations." *American Journal of Human Genetics* 67, no. 1: 170–81.

Reinarman, Craig, and Harry G. Levine. 1997. "The Crack Attack: Politics and Media in the Crack Scare." In *Crack in America: Demon Drugs and Social Justice*, edited by Craig Reinarman and Harry G. Levine, 18–51. Berkeley: University of California Press.

Rauner, Bruce. 2017. "State of Illinois Opioid Action Plan." dph.illinois.gov/sites/default/files/publications/Illinois-Opioid-Action-Plan-Sept-6-2017-FINAL.pdf (accessed October 21, 2019).

Scheufele, Dietram A., and David Tewksbury. 2007. "Framing, Agenda Setting, and Priming: The Evolution of Three Media Effects Models." *Journal of Communication* 57, no. 1: 9–20.

Sharpton, Al. 2018. "America's Racist Response to the Crack Epidemic Must Inform the Way We Tackle Opioids." NBC News, January 30. www.nbcnews.com/think/opinion/america-s-racist-response-crack-epidemic-must-inform-way-we-ncna842426.

Soleimani, Hossein, and David J. Miller. 2014. "Parsimonious Topic Models with Salient Word Discovery." *IEEE Transactions on Knowledge and Data Engineering* 27, no. 3: 824–37.

Unick, George Jay, Daniel Rosenblum, Sarah Mars, and Daniel Ciccarone. 2013. "Intertwined Epidemics: National Demographic Trends in Hospitalizations for Heroin- and Opioid-Related Overdoses, 1993–2009." *PLoS ONE* 8, no. 2: e54496.

Winter, Nicholas. 2006. "Beyond Welfare: Framing and the Racialization of White Opinion on Social Security." *American Journal of Political Science* 50, no. 2: 400–20.

Appendix A Analysis of Combined Opioid and Heroin Coverage in 2016–17

Unigrams

Rank	Word	Frequency
1	drug	22675
2	people	16878
3	health	15428
4	heroin	13609
5	opioid	12950
6	police	12544
7	drugs	10523
8	addiction	8623
9	care	8450
10	time	8446

Bigrams

Rank	Word	Word	Frequency
1	health	care	4186
2	public	health	2673
3	law	enforcement	2586
4	substance	abuse	2489
5	opioid	crisis	1853
6	dow	jones	1719
7	opioid	epidemic	1716
8	mental	health	1435
9	overdose	deaths	1353
10	white	house	1342

Trigrams

Rank	Word	Word	Word	Frequency
1	affordable	care	act	725
2	drug	enforcement	administration	557
3	health	care	reform	463
4	public	health	administration	443
5	controlled	substances	crime	442
6	substance	abuse	treatment	433
7	law	enforcement	officials	394
8	health	care	professionals	382
9	health	care	policy	370
10	health	care	law	359

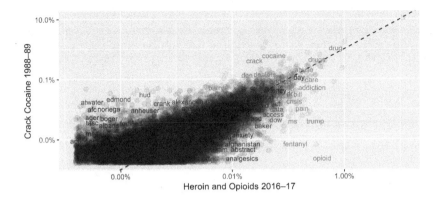

Appendix A Figure 1 Opioids (including heroin 2016–17) vs. crack cocaine, 1988–89.

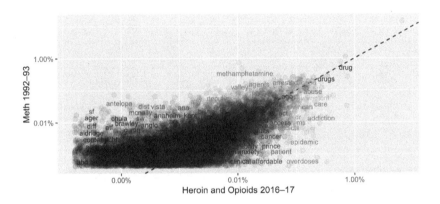

Appendix A Figure 2 Opioids (including heroin 2016–17) vs. methamphetamine, 1992–93.

Framing the Opioid Crisis: Do Racial Frames Shape Beliefs of Whites Losing Ground?

Sarah E. Gollust
University of Minnesota

Joanne M. Miller
University of Delaware

Abstract

Context: Although research has begun to examine perceptions of being on the losing side of politics, it has been confined to electoral politics. The context of health disparities, and particularly the opioid crisis, offers a case to explore whether frames that emphasize racial disadvantage activate loser perceptions and the political consequences of such beliefs.

Methods: White survey participants (N = 1,549) were randomized into three groups: a control which saw no news article, or one of two treatment groups which saw a news article about the opioid crisis framed to emphasize either the absolute rates of opioid mortality among whites or the comparative rates of opioid mortality among whites compared to blacks.

Findings: Among control group participants, perceiving oneself a political loser was unrelated to attitudes about addressing opioids, whereas those who perceived whites to be on the losing side of public health had a less empathetic response to the opioid crisis. The comparative frame led to greater beliefs that whites are on the losing side of public health, whereas the absolute frame led to more empathetic policy opinions.

Conclusions: Perceptions that one's racial group has lost ground in the public health context could have political consequences that future research should explore.

Keywords opioids, politics, media, public opinion

In a March 2018 survey by the Pew Research Center, a substantial majority of the public (67%; 78% of Democrats and 53% of Republicans) noted that "their side" has been losing more often than winning in politics. Given the high prevalence of this loser perception across both political parties (even among those whose party, at the time of the survey, controlled all three branches of the federal government), it is surprising that social

Journal of Health Politics, Policy and Law, Vol. 45, No. 2, April 2020
DOI 10.1215/03616878-8004874 © 2020 by Duke University Press

scientists actually know very little about the antecedents or consequences of these perceptions. In particular, little research attention has been paid to the factors that influence perceptions of being on the losing side of politics (or the consequences of such beliefs), nor has existing work explored the causes or consequences of perceptions of being on the losing side in specific policy domains. In the domain of public health policy, the notion of winners and losers is often quite explicit. For instance, certain groups are commonly portrayed as more or less affected by some conditions over others or there may be more policy attention (or funding) to one disease over another (Armstrong, Carpenter, and Hojnacki 2006; Best 2012). The consequences of these loser messages may be significant if perceptions of being advantaged versus disadvantaged contribute toward support for policies that have genuine potential to help or harm people's health. Whereas a few studies have examined public opinion about health disparities (Benz et al. 2011; Booske, Robert, and Rohan 2011), this literature in public health has been disconnected from the literature in political psychology explaining the psychological predispositions of policy beliefs. The current study aims to bridge these literatures and offer new insights into the political consequences of believing oneself to be on the losing side of public health policy, focusing on opioid use disorder (OUD) as a case wherein these phenomena may be particularly salient. Elite messaging around OUD has often portrayed the problem as being particularly severe among white Americans, potentially activating the types of loser sentiments described above.

The objectives of this research are to examine the factors that predict whites' perceptions of being a loser both in politics and in health policy, assess whether such perceptions have an impact on support for policies to address OUD, and test whether these loser perceptions can be manipulated by elite messaging about the racialized demographics of the opioid crisis. There are two potential classes of policy responses to the opioid problem, one that is more empathetic of people with OUD (i.e., bolstering public health approaches of treatment and prevention while reducing stigma) and another that is more punitive (i.e., focusing on drug use and its correlates as crimes among users, dealers, and inappropriate prescribers). Identifying what factors predict the public's support for these positions thus provides important contributions to the evolving policy response to the crisis. The study also contributes to theory in two ways. First, we demonstrate that loser perceptions have consequences for policy attitudes in the domain of opioid policy, and they are not explained away by the usual predictors of political attitudes like demographics and partisanship. Second, we show that loser perceptions can be manipulated by elite messages. Although the magnitude of the findings are small, we anticipate that these propositions will foster additional scholarship into the political consequences of a type of elite messaging that situates one group as winning and another as losing—messaging that is extremely common in both current politics and public health, as we describe below.

Background on the Political Psychology of the Loser

With the recent rise in populism, support for so-called populist candidates (such as Donald Trump), ethnocentrism, and anti-immigrant attitudes—especially among whites—has come an increase in scholarly attention to the role of concepts such as alienation, efficacy, and economic, cultural, and racial threat in affecting individuals' political attitudes and behaviors. For example, journalists and scholars alike have used individual- and community-level data to examine the causes of whites' support for Donald Trump, oftentimes in an attempt to disentangle the effects of racial, economic, and cultural threat (or to argue that one was more impactful than the others; see, e.g., Chokshi 2018). In *White Identity Politics*, Ashley Jardina (2019) argues that the perception that the United States is losing ground culturally, sparked by growing diversity in the country, is a primary determinant of support for policies and candidates that whites (especially those who strongly identify with their racial group) believe will "Make America Great Again." In *Dying of Whiteness*, Jonathan Metzl (2019) argues that whites' investment in policies that contribute toward maintenance of racial superiority harms their own health and well-being. As he notes, "White backlash politics gave certain white populations the sensation of *winning* (emphasis added), particularly by upending the gains of minorities and liberals; yet the victories came at steep cost," the cost of their own health (Metzl 2019: 8). At the root of these explanations is the notion that a dominant group's belief that they are losing ground is fundamental to our understanding of the rise of populist sentiments and ethnocentrism around the globe (Cramer 2016 makes a similar argument with regard to rural white Americans).

Research narrowly targeted on the consequences of the political psychology of losing is limited. Miller, Farhart, and Saunders (2018) have shown that people who perceive themselves to be on the losing side of politics are more likely to endorse conspiracy theories that impugn their political rivals and that the perceived threat of losing power is causally related to reduced support for political compromise (Barker, Bowler,

Carman, and Wendelbo 2018). Other work shows that people who vote for the losing presidential candidate become less trusting of government (Anderson and LoTempio 2002; see also Nadeau and Blais 1993) and that electoral losers are more likely to believe in election fraud conspiracies than electoral winners (e.g., Edelson et al. 2017). Researchers have also shown that learned helplessness—a concept related to perceiving oneself a loser—is negatively correlated with conventional forms of political participation (e.g., voting) and positively correlated to unconventional participation (e.g., protesting), especially among traditionally disadvantaged racial minorities (Farhart 2017).

The perception that one, or one's group, is on the losing side (of politics, or of a particular policy domain) is also similar to one component of the psychological concept of relative deprivation. People naturally compare themselves, and their outcomes, with others (either as individuals comparing themselves to other individuals—egoistic relative deprivation—or as members of a group comparing themselves to members of other groups—fraternal or group relative deprivation; Runciman 1993). To the extent that people notice others possess something to which they feel entitled and think is feasible to obtain, and do not blame themselves for failure to possess it, resentment results (Crosby 1976). Our conceptualization of loser perceptions is akin to the first component of group level relative deprivation—the realization that another group possesses something that one's own group does not possess (e.g., the perception that one's political party is on the losing side of politics, or one's racial group is on the losing side of health policy).

The two domains in which the effects of relative deprivation have been most examined are worker satisfaction with their pay/income inequality (e.g., Sweeney, McFarlin, and Inderrieden 1990) and political protest and social movement participation (e.g., Pettigrew 2015; Smith and Huo 2014). Relative deprivation has been linked to a host of emotional and behavioral effects, such as objective and subjective (decreases in) happiness, depression, health, satisfaction with one's job and salary, aggression, and social movement participation (e.g., Subramanyam et al. 2009; but see Gurney and Tierney 1982 for a critique of the application of relative deprivation theory to social movements). Interestingly, although the theory of relative deprivation has been applied to make policy recommendations surrounding issues of pay equity, income inequality, social justice, and the like (Smith and Huo 2014), to our knowledge, research has not explored the *policy attitudes* of individuals who are experiencing relative deprivation. Moreover, little work has examined the causes and political consequences of perceptions that one's group is on the losing side of politics in general or within specific policy domains (although see Metzl 2019 for an example). As such, we focus in this study on the causes and policy attitude consequences of group-level loser perceptions.

Background on Framing Health Disparities

Health disparities in the United States is one policy domain for which the concept of group-level loser perceptions may be particularly salient. Health disparities are defined as differences in health that "adversely affect socially disadvantaged groups; are systematic and plausibly avoidable" (Braveman et al. 2011). Research consistently shows that populations that face structural inequality (e.g., lower socioeconomic status, residential segregation, or racism) also experience disproportionate rates of illness (Braveman et al. 2011). Whereas the public health literature abounds with discussion of health disparities, understanding of health inequalities among the public is more limited. For instance, in 2010, only 45% of Americans were aware that African Americans have worse life expectancy than whites; 37% were aware that African Americans are more likely than whites to be diagnosed with diabetes (Benz et al. 2011). Low public awareness may result from a news media that comments infrequently about health disparities in typical health coverage (Gollust and Lantz 2009; Nagler et al. 2016).

Elite messaging—or framing—has the potential to shift public views on health disparities. Framing is the strategic emphasis communicators place on certain aspects of social or political issues, such as the causes, solutions, or target populations affected, in public or media discourse (Entman 1993). Research on framing, for instance, demonstrates that emphasizing the racial identity of a group affected by public policy can shape public attitudes about those issues (see, e.g., Kinder and Sanders 1996).[1] Relatively few studies have sought to understand how framing group-level health disparities affects public understanding (see Niederdeppe et al. 2013 for a review). In one study that explicitly examines social comparison frames (i.e., presenting racial comparisons of illness risk as opposed to reporting a single group's risk), Bigman (2014) found that comparative frames tended to

1. Another broad class of literature on framing in health communication concerns loss or gain frames (Rothman et al. 2006). Whereas the idea of a loss frame is conceptually related to the idea of being a loser, loss-framed messages in the health communication context are typically messages that identify the costs of not taking some protective action to reduce one's health risk versus a gain-framed message, which identifies the health benefits of taking the action. Since these frames are typically focused on individualized health behavior choices (and not group issues or policy preferences), these frames are not our focus here.

decrease perceptions of risk for the less at-risk group. In another experimental study, Nicholson and colleagues (2008) found that a frame describing blacks as having higher colon cancer rates led to black respondents having negative reactions and lowered colorectal cancer screening intentions. Neither of these studies included politically relevant outcome measures, however, such as support for policy. Gollust and Cappella (2014) tested various messages describing the causes of disparities between socioeconomic groups and found high levels of anger elicitation and counterarguing in response to the messages; conservative respondents counterargued the messages more than liberals did. This study suggests that disparity frames could produce politically consequential responses, either because they activate motivated reasoning (i.e., the motivation to challenge the very existence of disparities or the need for government to address them) or other types of racialized stereotypes (Kinder and Sanders 1996), such as minority racial groups being to blame for their disadvantaged status (Lynch and Gollust 2010). However, no work to our knowledge has examined whether framing disparities in health outcomes might contribute toward the political psychology of feeling like a loser or whether such a perception has broader political consequences.

Opioid Use Disorder as a Case

The opioid crisis is a salient case in which to explore the political psychology of health disparities frames and the effect of loser perceptions on policy attitudes. Opioid use disorder (OUD) generally concerns problematic use of prescription pain medications and/or heroin or street versions of synthetic opiates like fentanyl. The opioid case offers a different perspective from how scholars traditionally understand health disparity. In national depictions of the opioid problem, the racial group typically perceived as more advantaged in US society — whites — is suffering (in terms of higher levels of addiction and overdose mortality based on national statistics), more than those groups typically perceived as disadvantaged (i.e., people of color; see Hansen and Netherland 2016). For instance, there were 37,113 total deaths from overdoses among whites in 2017 (a rate of 19.4 per 100,000) compared to 5,513 deaths among blacks (a rate of 12.9 per 100,000; KFF n.d.).[2]

2. Recent health data document accelerating rates of OUD among all population groups, with particularly steep increases among Native American and urban African American populations, especially low-income African Americans in certain metropolitan areas such as Washington, DC (CDC 2018; Jamison 2018).

This population comparative frame—emphasizing high rates among whites compared to other groups—is featured prominently in news coverage of OUD (Harbin 2019; Netherland and Hansen 2016; see also Shachar et al., this issue). For example, a May 2018 *New York Times Magazine* cover article reported on the higher prevalence of neonatal abstinence syndrome among whites and featured numerous anecdotes and photographs of white mothers and babies. The author even reflectively noted in her coverage, "Indeed, the perception of our opioid crisis as an *epidemic*, rather than a racial pathology, owes much to the fact that white Americans have been hard hit" (Egan 2018).

This novel disparity frame has also been the subject of scholarly interest. Health disparities researchers have questioned whether the dissemination of the concept of working-class white mortality from addiction and related mental health conditions will contribute toward public perceptions of a "new face of disadvantage," despite the enduring health inequities for communities of color (Brown and Tucker-Seeley 2018: 124). At the core of our current research are similar questions: Do common racialized media frames of opioid use disorder promote whites' perception that they are losers in public health? And what are the consequences of such beliefs on attitudes about policy and resource allocation?

Understanding the consequences of loser perceptions surrounding the opioid crisis is significant for several reasons. First, a growing research narrative links whites' morbidity and mortality from overdose, suicide, and mental illness (see, e.g., Case and Deaton 2015) to voting in the 2016 election. Several recent studies identify correlations at the ecological level between poor community health (including addiction) and whites' turnout for Trump in 2016 (Bor 2017; Monnat and Brown 2017; Wasfy, Stewart III, and Bhambhani 2017). If racial comparison frames emphasizing white opioid threats activate perceptions that whites are losing, this could be politically consequential. For instance, emphasizing this losing status could boost whites' support of government spending on opioids—but it could potentially lower their support for spending on illnesses more common among nonwhites.

Second, framing the opioid crisis as a "white issue" could lead whites to be more sympathetic toward opioid users than they would otherwise be (in comparison to drug use problems that plague communities of color, as noted in the popular press; see, e.g., Lopez 2017). Policy responses to high rates of OUD might be categorized into an *empathetic* approach that favors public health policy strategies and a *punitive* approach that emphasizes law enforcement strategies (McGinty et al. 2016; see also Kim, Morgan, and

Nyhan in this issue). The former includes public health education, treatment with effective pharmacological remedies (i.e., medically assisted treatment), guidelines to promote more appropriate opioid prescribing by providers, and harm reduction approaches (such as treatment of overdose with naloxone and needle exchange; Barry et al. 2016; Saloner and Barry 2018). Punitive approaches include arresting and prosecuting those who possess, use, or deal opioids, cracking down on providers and clinics that are unlawfully prescribing opioids, enforcing immigration laws to prevent the trafficking of drugs, and referring parents or pregnant women who use drugs to child welfare authorities (Kennedy-Hendricks et al. 2017). Loser perceptions could lead members of the public (and policy makers alike) to favor different types of empathetic versus punitive policies as appropriate responses to the opioid crisis (Kennedy-Hendricks et al. 2017).

Research Objectives

This study has two major objectives. First, given the paucity of research on the political consequences of perceiving oneself to be a political loser, we examine the correlates, predictors of, and consequences of feeling like a loser in politics (among a sample of white Americans *not* exposed to news frames about the opioid crisis). We also develop a measure to assess the belief that whites are on the losing side of public health policy, and compare the correlates, predictors of, and consequences of health loser perceptions with political loser perceptions. Specifically, we assess whether loser perceptions are related to public attitudes about the appropriate approaches to deal with the opioid epidemic. Second, using an experiment, we examine whether frames that emphasize white mortality (in either an absolute or a comparative sense) affect whites' propensity to identify as a loser in the political context or the health context, as well as whether these frames affect public support for policy approaches.

Our study design is guided by a general conceptual model (see figure 1). The model proposes that *loser perceptions*—perceiving oneself on the losing side of politics or policy—may contribute to *policy-relevant attitudes* about an issue (i.e., empathetic vs. punitive policy approaches and attitudes about the target population). Examining the factors that are associated with loser perceptions (both predictors of and consequences on policy-relevant outcomes) is the first task of the study, relying on the control group from our experiment. Leveraging an embedded media framing experiment, we further anticipate that *media frames* describing white opioid mortality using a comparative frame (i.e., explicitly stating that whites have higher rates of opioid mortality than blacks) will activate perceptions

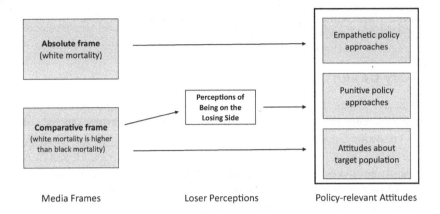

Figure 1 Stylized model of relationships tested in the study.

of being on the losing side more than the same article with an absolute frame (i.e., just reporting opioid mortality rates among whites). We also explore whether these frames have effects on policy-relevant attitudes—directly or via loser perceptions.

Data and Methods

Data were collected through Amazon Mechanical Turk (MTurk) on August 3, 2018. MTurk provides access to more demographically diverse samples of the US voting-age population than student-convenience and Internet samples (Berinsky, Huber, and Lenz 2012; Buhrmester, Kwang, and Gosling 2011; Levay, Freese, and Druckman 2016), as well as high-quality data (Crump, McDonnell, and Gureckis 2013; Goodman, Cryder, and Cheema 2013; Weinberg, Freese, and McElhattan 2014). After eliminating 124 respondents we suspected to be bots, there were 1953 participants in the study.[3] Given our theoretical expectations that the messages

3. A concern has arisen among scholars who use MTurk that there has been a substantial uptick (since spring 2018) in the number of responses submitted from identical GPS coordinates (possibly completed by bots). Anecdotal evidence from scholars' social media conversations indicates that between 5% and 50% of recently collected MTurk survey responses come from repeating GPS coordinates. Some repeating GPS coordinates are to be expected (www.qualtrics .com/support/survey-platform/data-and-analysis-module/data/download-data/understanding -your-dataset/), and the bot problem may be not as pervasive as the social media discussions among academics make it out to be (blog.turkprime.com/2018/08/concerns-about-bots-on -mechanical-turk.html?m=1). We erred on the side of caution by dropping from our data any response that had the same GPS coordinates as at least nine other responses (29 with GPS coordinates that put them in a reservoir in Kansas, 39 from a park in Buffalo, NY, and 13 from the same GPS coordinates in Venezuela).

would affect whites' beliefs specifically, we restrict all analyses to adults who identify as white (N = 1,549).

Study Design

After answering questions about their interest in news and politics, participants were randomly assigned to one of three conditions. In two of the conditions, participants viewed a news article about the opioid crisis. They were told, "A new report from Trust for America's Health was recently published about the state of public health in America. Please read the following news article about the report and answer the questions that follow." Participants in the absolute frame condition (N = 510) saw an article titled "Rising Opioid Addictions Pose a Threat to Health of White Americans" that presented data (along with a figure) about the high rates of opioid overdose mortality rates among whites. Participants in the comparative frame condition (N = 504) saw an article entitled "Rising Opioid Addictions Pose a Greater Threat to Health of White Americans than Black Americans" that presented data (along with a figure) about the differential rates of opioid overdose mortality rates between whites and blacks (see appendix 1 for full text of articles). Participants in the third condition (control group) received no article and completed the rest of the survey. This group (N = 535) was used in the first set of (nonexperimental) analyses.

Participants in the treatment conditions were asked three questions to assess their opinions about the article (how interesting/informative they perceived it to be, and how likely they would be to share it, measured on Likert scales coded 1 = not at all, 2 = slightly, 3 = somewhat, 4 = very, and 5 = extremely) before answering additional survey items that the no-exposure control group also answered.

Manipulation Check. To test whether the two articles were effective at communicating that the rates of opioid addiction are higher among whites, all respondents were asked a question adapted from previous research assessing public awareness of health disparities (Benz et al. 2011): "Compared to the average white person, do you think the average African American person is more likely, just as likely, or less likely to be affected by . . . " [opioid addiction]. The response options were coded such that 1 = less likely, 2 = just as likely, and 3 = more likely. This question was asked following the news article and the loser perception questions.

Loser Status. The general loser perception question, based on a question adapted from the Pew Research Center (Fingerhut 2015) by Miller,

Farhart, and Saunders (2018) asked, "Thinking about the way things are going in politics today, *on the issues that matter to you*, would you say that your side has been winning more often than it's been losing, or losing more often than it's been winning?" Response options were "winning more often than losing" and "losing more often than winning" which branched to a second question. The second question asked, "Would you say that your side is winning [losing]?" and response options included "a great deal more often than losing [winning]," "somewhat more often than losing [winning]," or "a little bit more than losing [winning]." These questions were combined to create a 6-point scale, with higher numbers representing greater loser perceptions.

We also created a health policy-specific loser perception measure.[4] Given that one of our goals was to examine whether the correlates and consequences of health loser perceptions are similar to general political loser perceptions, we constructed this question to be as similar as possible to the Pew question. However, rather than using the language of "your *side*," we chose to highlight a racial group comparison, to tap the kinds of comparisons that are frequently made in the health policy domain. Respondents were asked, "Thinking about the way things are going with the public's health, do you think that *white* Americans are on the winning side or the losing side of public policies aimed at improving health outcomes compared to *black* Americans?" As with the general political loser question, the winning/losing question was then branched to a follow-up question, which asked, "Would you say that white Americans are winning [losing]" "a great deal more often than losing [winning]," "somewhat more often than losing [winning]," or "a little bit more than losing [winning]." These questions were combined to create a 6-point scale, with higher numbers representing greater loser perceptions. We chose not to include a middle option because neither the original Pew item nor Miller et al.'s (2018) branched version did so.

---

4. Given the limited research examining loser status in health or politics, we first fielded a pilot study from September 27 to October 5, 2017, also using an MTurk sample of whites only. In this survey we piloted a few other items assessing dimensions of being a loser in public health, including a dichotomous version of the measure described above (winning vs. losing) along with the political loser status item and a smaller number of opioid policy opinions. To assess the validity of the key measures, we compared the predictors of the political loser and public health loser items in both the 2017 and 2018 surveys. A comparison of the 2017 pilot with the 2018 survey provides substantial evidence that the items are measuring similar underlying concepts despite different samples and different times of data collection (results available from authors upon request).

Policy Opinions. We assessed attitudes toward a set of 12 policy proposals, adapted from previous work (Barry et al. 2016; see appendix 2 for the full set, as well as the means from the control group). The items were selected based on whether they would be considered empathetic or punitive responses toward people with OUD (and/or their health care providers). Response options were coded such that 1 = strongly oppose, 2 = oppose, 3 = somewhat oppose, 4 = neither favor nor oppose, 5 = somewhat favor, 6 = favor, and 7 = strongly favor. These items, and all other policy items described below, were displayed in random order. We constructed scales from these items based on whether they were public health–oriented (empathetic) measures or law-enforcement (punitive) measures. The empathetic policy opinion scale (alpha = .84) is an average of the first six items listed in appendix 2. The punitive policy opinion scale (alpha = .80) is an average of the second six items.

Government Spending. Respondents were asked whether they thought the government should spend more or less on the following three empathetic domains: treatment for opioid addiction, drug overdose prevention programs, and education campaigns about the dangers of opioid addiction; and the following two punitive domains: law enforcement to arrest opioid dealers and opioid users, respectively. All responses were measured on a 5-point scale such that 1 = spend much less, 2 = spend less, 3 = spend about the same, 4 = spend more, and 5 = spend a lot more.

Responsibility. Respondents were asked how much responsibility they thought "the following groups should have for addressing the problem of opioid (prescription pain medication and heroin) abuse in the United States" (adapted from Barry et al. 2016): pharmacies and pharmacists, pharmaceutical companies, doctors, and health insurance companies (averaged to comprise a health care industry responsibility scale with an alpha of .81), the federal government (we treated these two groups as empathetic), dealers, addicts, and law enforcement (we treated these latter three groups as punitive). Responses were coded such that 1 = none, 2 = a little, 3 = a moderate amount, 4 = a lot, and 5 = a great deal.

Attitudes toward People with Opioid Addiction. We used a standard 0–100 feeling thermometer measure to assess attitudes toward people with opioid addiction (McGinty et al. 2018). In addition to people who abuse opioids (mean in control condition = 45.6), participants were asked about people who have been diagnosed with depression (mean = 75.0), people who abuse alcohol (mean = 47.3), people who have been diagnosed with HIV (mean = 65.0), and people who have been diagnosed with cancer (mean = 80.8).[5] Not surprisingly, respondents reported feeling the coldest toward people whose afflictions are perceived to be more in their control (those who abuse opioids and alcohol, as well as people diagnosed with HIV), with those who abuse opioids garnering the most negative rating (Weiner 2006).

Spending on Other Health Disparities. To assess whether the frames might have a negative effect on people's support for government spending to prevent health problems more prevalent among black Americans, respondents were asked, "Do you think the federal government spends too much money, spends the right amount of money, or spends too little money on programs aimed at preventing health problems that are more prevalent among *black* Americans compared to *white* Americans?" Responses were coded such that 1 = spends too much money, 2 = spends enough money, and 3 = spends too little money.

Control Variables. We measured the following political and demographic variables: party identification, gender, annual income, age, education, Hispanic/Latinx ethnicity, strength of white identity, and respondents' subjective perceptions of their relative socioeconomic status (see appendix 3 for the question wordings and coding for these variables).

Analysis

In the first set of analyses, we focused only on the white respondents in the control condition to examine the distributions of the two loser perception variables (political and health policy), as well as their correlations. Next, we examined the factors that predict these loser perceptions, by regressing each of the two loser perception variables on the set of sociodemographic and political characteristics using ordinary least squares (OLS) regression. Third, to assess the political consequences of these perceptions, we regressed the three sets of responses to the opioid crisis as dependent variables (empathetic policy attitudes, punitive policy attitudes, and stigma held toward users) on the two loser perception variables and included the same set of sociodemographic and political controls.

---

5. We note that our survey wording used the language of abuse in response to the problem and in assessing stigma toward people who use drugs and alcohol, which we acknowledge is problematic and can itself perpetuate stigma. Thus, in this article we used the word abuse in reference to the survey language respondents saw and otherwise used opioid use disorder and other nonstigmatizing language elsewhere. See, for example, "Words Matter: How Language Choice Can Reduce Stigma," Substance Abuse and Mental Health Services Administration (SAMHSA), mnprc.org/2017/02/04/words-matter-how-language-choice-can-reduce-stigma/ (accessed November 12, 2019).

For the experimental analyses, we first verified that respondents were balanced in observable characteristics (the control variables described above) across the three experimental groups, using linear regression and chi-square tests. We observed no significant differences across the randomly assigned groups in these characteristics. We used t-tests and chi-square tests to assess whether there were any differences between the two treatment groups (absolute vs. comparative racial framing) in responses to the knowledge question about rates of addiction by racial group (e.g., our manipulation check) and in evaluations of the news vignettes (how interesting, shareable, and informative they were).

To assess whether there were differences in loser perceptions and in participants' responses to the opioid epidemic by the experimental frame to which they were exposed, we regressed the three sets of dependent variables (loser perceptions, policy attitudes, feeling thermometer) on the treatment groups. We estimated the regression models with and without covariates to assess whether inclusion of control variables affected the precision of our experimental estimates. We used postestimation Wald tests of the coefficients on the experimental conditions to test for differences between conditions.

Results

Nonexperimental Results (Control Condition Only)

Table 1 displays the characteristics of the group without exposure to any opioid news story (white respondents only). The sample is reasonably varied in terms of socioeconomic status and partisanship, but as is typical of MTurk samples, it is more Democratic, younger, and more educated than the US adult population as a whole.

Participants more readily acknowledged feeling like they are on the losing side with regard to politics than they acknowledged that white Americans are on the losing side with regard to health policy. Specifically, the mean of the political loser measure (6-point scale ranging from winning a lot more to losing a lot more) was 3.64 (SD = 1.73), whereas the mean of the racialized health policy loser measure was 2.47 (SD = 1.4). Over half (51.9%) of respondents reported that they believed they were losing a little, somewhat, or a lot more than winning in politics. In contrast, only 18.6% of respondents reported that white Americans were losing a little, somewhat, or a lot more than they were winning in health policy.

Relationship between Political and Health Policy Loser Status. The political loser and the health policy loser variables were uncorrelated ($r = -.05$, ns). The fact that the political loser question asks respondents to indicate whether they think their side is losing [winning] more often than winning [losing] (likely activating partisanship and/or political ideology), whereas the health policy loser question explicitly asks respondents whether they think white Americans are losing [winning] more often than winning [losing] in the health policy domain *relative to black Americans*, may be one of the reasons for a lack of association between the two. Consistent with this reasoning (and unsurprisingly given that at the time of the survey Republicans controlled both the executive and legislative branches of the federal government), Democrats scored *higher* on the political loser variable than Republicans (means = 4.46 and 2.51, respectively, $t = 14.49$, $p < .001$). In contrast, Democrats scored *lower* on the explicitly racialized health policy loser variable than Republicans (means = 2.11 and 2.76, respectively, $t = -5.24$, $p < .001$).

Predictors of Loser Status. Before running OLS regressions to examine the predictors of political and health loser perceptions, we recoded all variables (independent and dependent) to range from 0–1. Table 2 displays the factors that predict loser perceptions. Men, Republicans, political conservatives, those with a bachelor's degree or some college (compared to more than a college education), and those reporting their social standing was high were all significantly *less* likely to report being a loser in the domain of politics, while those over age 50 were *more* likely to report being a political loser. Those with a stronger white racial identity were also significantly less likely to report being a political loser. These findings have strong face validity, illuminating the groups who arguably were achieving more wins than losses in politics during the summer of 2018, before the fall electoral victories of women, people of color, and Democrats.

The pattern of predictors was different for the racialized health policy loser variable. Whites who were older, Independent, and politically conservative were more likely to perceive whites to be on the losing side of health policy. Those who reported a higher social standing were *less* likely to perceive whites to be on the losing side of health policy. In fact, those who reported a higher social standing were significantly less likely to endorse being on the losing side of *both* politics and health policy, reinforcing the validity of these measures. Interestingly, despite the racially explicit nature of the health policy loser variable, strength of white identity had no relationship to respondents' belief that whites are health policy losers.

Consequences of Loser Perceptions on Opioid Policy Attitudes. For these loser perceptions to be politically consequential, they need to be related to policy attitudes. Table 3 reports the results of separate OLS regression models predicting the empathetic and punitive attitudes, as well as the stigma measure, with both the political and health loser perception variables in models that include the controls (all independent and dependent variables were recoded to range from 0–1; full models are available from the authors upon request). Political loser status was associated with three of the empathetic attitudes and two of the punitive policy attitudes (and inconsistently so); political loser perception was negatively associated with the punitive policy index (b = −.11, p < .001) and positively associated with the belief that dealers are responsible (b = .15, p < .001). It was not associated with the stigma measure.

Results for the health policy loser status question are more consistent. The perception that white Americans are on the losing side in health policy is negatively associated with every one of the empathetic attitudes, and is not associated with any of the punitive attitudes or the feeling thermometer. Whites who perceive that they are on the losing side of public policies aimed at improving health outcomes compared to blacks are *less* supportive of policies and government spending programs that are empathetic to opioid users, and believe that the health care sector and the federal government are *less* responsible for addressing the problem compared to whites who perceive that they are on the winning side.

Experimental Results

Manipulation Check. To examine whether the articles were effective at communicating to respondents that opioid addiction rates are higher among whites, we examined the percentage of respondents in each condition who said that African Americans are less likely to be affected by opioid addiction. Compared to the control condition (16%), more respondents in the absolute (27%) and comparative (49%) conditions indicated that African Americans are less affected (from logistic regression, b = .71, se = .15 and b = 1.64, se = .15 for the absolute and comparative conditions respectively compared to the no-exposure control condition, p < .05). Although the effect of the manipulation was not very strong, those exposed to the treatment conditions were more accurate in their assessments that African Americans were less likely to be affected by opioid addiction than respondents in the control condition, and they were most accurate when provided the explicit comparative frame in the article.

In addition, respondents in the absolute (mean = 2.31) and comparative (mean = 2.37) conditions were equally likely to indicate that they would share the article with friends or family if they were to see the article online (t = .78, ns). Respondents in the comparative condition were significantly more likely to indicate that they found the article to be interesting (means = 3.49 and 3.37, respectively, t = 1.98, p < .05) and marginally significantly more likely to indicate that they found the article to be informative (means = 3.67 and 3.57, respectively, t = 1.74, p < .10).

Effect of the Frames on Loser Perceptions. We tested our hypothesis that the comparative frame would be more likely to activate loser perceptions than the absolute frame (compared to the control) by regressing the political loser question, and then the health policy loser question, on the two treatment dummy variables. As table 4 shows, consistent with expectations, the respondents in the absolute condition were no more likely to perceive themselves to be on the losing side of politics, nor that whites are on the losing side of health policies, than respondents in the no-exposure condition. However, respondents in the comparative frame condition were more likely to perceive whites to be on the losing side in the health domain compared to respondents in the no-exposure condition (b = .03, p < .10 in the model without control variables; b = .04, p < .05 in the model with control variables). The effect of the comparative condition on perceptions of being a political loser was not statistically significant.

Thus far, we have shown the perception that whites are losing ground to blacks in the health policy domain is powerfully, and *negatively*, associated with empathetic opioid attitudes, and that the comparative frame is predictive of this belief that whites are losing ground. Next, we turn to examining the impact of the frames on opioid attitudes.

Effect of the Frames on Opioid Attitudes. Results of the effects of the frames relative to the control on the punitive policy measure and the empathetic policy measure are shown in table 5. Specifically, participants in the absolute condition were significantly more likely to support empathetic policies (b = .03, p < .01 in the model without controls; b = .04, p < .001 in the model with controls) compared to those in the no-exposure condition. Participants in the comparative condition were marginally significantly more likely to support empathetic policies (b = 02, p < .10) compared to the no-exposure condition, but only in the model without controls. However, we could not reject the null hypothesis of no difference between the absolute condition and comparative condition in their impact on support for empathetic policies (Wald test F = 1.20, p = .274). The treatment conditions had no impact on support for punitive policies, relative to the no-exposure condition.

Neither of the treatment conditions had statistically significant effects (at $p < 0.05$) on any of the other policy attitudes examined (responsibility attributions or government spending), nor on the feeling thermometer measure of stigma (results available upon request).

To review the key experimental findings, we identified that the comparative frame led to greater perceptions of whites' being on the losing side of health policy, and that in the control condition perceptions of being on the losing side of health policy were associated with lower support for empathetic policies. In contrast, we found that the absolute frame led to greater support for empathetic policies, and minimal evidence that the comparative frame had any impact on policy attitudes at all. Given these conflicting findings, we have no conceptual evidence for the mediation path depicted in figure 1, that any effect of the comparative frame on policy-relevant attitudes is indirect, via loser perceptions.[6]

Effect of the Frames on Health Disparity Spending. The final goal of the analysis was to evaluate whether there may be any negative consequences of the emphasis of white Americans as having a high rate of opioid mortality on perceptions of other racial health disparities. Collapsing across the three conditions, 9.6% of respondents indicated that they thought that the government spends too much money on health problems more prevalent among black Americans compared to white Americans; 47.3% of respondents indicated that the government spent enough money, and 43.2% indicated that the government spends too little money. There were no significant differences across the treatment groups in the belief that the government spends too much money on health problems among blacks ($\chi^2 = 4.61$, ns), indicating that the treatment conditions did not cause a backlash on support for spending on other health disparities.

Discussion

This study aimed to identify whether perceptions of feeling like a loser in health politics might be politically consequential, and whether certain ways of framing racial disparities for one issue—the opioid epidemic—might affect such perceptions. The results are mixed but offer new insights into the politics of the opioid epidemic as well as suggest new lines of

6. We also tested a simple mediation model with regression analysis and found no statistical support that loser perceptions mediate the effects of the experimental frames on policy attitudes. However, we acknowledge that analyses attempting to apply a causal interpretation to cross-sectional mediation analyses have challenges related to confounding (see, e.g., MacKinnon and Pirlott 2015).

inquiry within the broad intersection of political psychology and health disparity research in public health.

We measured two constructs, the status of whites' perceiving themselves to be a loser in politics (endorsed by a majority of the sample, as with the Pew 2018 survey) and in a racialized health policy domain (endorsed by only 1 in 5 respondents). We found that these beliefs are uncorrelated with one another, yet are systematically related to other sociodemographic and political characteristics in ways that support the validity of these items. Namely, whites in 2018 who were conservative, Republican, and identified more strongly with their white identity were less likely to feel like a political loser. In contrast, conservatives were more likely to feel whites were losing in the health policy domain. Importantly, the higher respondents perceived themselves on the ladder of subjective social status, the less likely they were to perceive themselves a loser in either politics or in health policy, as one would expect.

These two beliefs predicted attitudes about opioids differently. The belief of being a loser in politics was largely unrelated to any opioid attitudes—on policy, spending, responsibility attributions, or stigma. In contrast, white respondents' perception that whites are on the losing side of public health policy was consistently and negatively related to empathetic approaches to deal with the opioid epidemic. Even when adjusting for demographic factors, partisanship, and ideology, this belief of whites being a loser in health policy was related to opposition toward a set of policies considered by public health authorities to be evidence-based ways to deal with the epidemic, including increasing access to treatment, naloxone availability, and education campaigns (Barry et al. 2016; Saloner and Barry 2018). Our findings suggest that this belief of whites being on the losing side—often discussed in terms of the 2016 election results—could be an important contributor to public health politics as well. As noted by others (Goodwin et al. 2018; Monnat and Brown 2017; Wasfy, Stewart III, and Bhambhani 2017), there may be a relationship between the extent of the opioid crisis and county-level voting patterns for Trump in 2016. If whites living in these areas also feel higher levels of being a loser in public health, they may be less supportive of the very policies that might best ameliorate the opioid crisis in their areas. And, if media frames continue to emphasize this perception of whites losing ground—as journalists have done in the past (Netherland and Hansen 2016), the media could contribute to reifying these beliefs—and consequently policy opinions—more strongly.

We found limited evidence to support the experimental expectations of the study: neither framing the opioid crisis to emphasize whites as the group affected, nor framing it to compare whites to blacks, had strong effects on either perceptions of whites' being a disadvantaged group in politics (null results only) or in health policy (small effects for the comparative condition). We did find that the absolute condition, which emphasized whites as the dominant group suffering from the opioid epidemic, led to stronger support for an empathic policy approach to deal with the epidemic but had very little effect on other beliefs about the epidemic.[7] The fact that the absolute framing of whites as the major population affected by opioids, relative to no exposure to any media depiction, did shape a more empathic response to the epidemic is broadly consistent with media commentary on the epidemic (see, e.g., Lopez 2017; also see Kim, Morgan, and Nyhan in this issue). In other words, emphasizing the white target population may contribute to a more empathetic policy approach to deal with the problem among a white audience. Finally, concerns of an unintended effect of framing white mortality in the opioid context—that it could drive down support for spending on conditions that are more common in nonwhite racial groups—were not borne out in these data.

Limitations and Future Directions

This study offers an initial exploration into the political consequences of losing ground in public health. Future work should continue to unpack the relationships between health loser perceptions and policy attitudes, recognizing that cross-sectional analyses have limitations. Our experimental and nonexperimental results together raise some questions we cannot completely unpack, such as why the comparative frame contributed toward whites' heightened perceptions of feeling like a loser but also increased support for empathetic policy responses, whereas whites' perception that their racial group is losing was negatively correlated with empathetic policy responses. There may be selection issues, confounding, and/or omitted variables that the current models cannot address.[8] We cannot, for

7. Per a suggestion by a workshop participant for this special issue, we also examined whether there was any heterogeneity in the effects of the frames across whites based on their measured strength of white identity. This variable was measured postrandomization so our post hoc assessment of interaction effects was exploratory (and we note that the frames had no effect on strength of white identity). We did not find any evidence that the frames had a significantly different effect on perceptions of whites being on the losing side of health policy or on policy attitudes among respondents who perceived their white identity to be weaker or stronger.

8. We attempted to examine endogeneity concerns in the relationship between loser status and policy attitudes with instrumental variables analysis, where random assignment to the comparative frame was an instrument for health loser perceptions (see, e.g., MacKinnon and Pirlott 2015). However, we do not believe the frames affected the outcome exclusively through loser perceptions, so the assumption for this analysis was not met. The first-stage F statistic was 4.11, much lower than conventional cut-offs to be considered a strong instrument, so these analyses were not conclusive.

instance, distinguish health loser perception (as measured here, with its explicit whites versus blacks comparison) from various types of racial resentment (Feldman and Huddy 2005; Jardina 2019; Kinder and Sanders 1996). The health loser perception question may be tapping the general belief that blacks get more than they deserve rather than the perception that whites are on the losing side in a specific public policy domain. Although we did show that strength of white identity was unrelated to health policy loser perceptions, future research should measure and explicitly control for racial resentment.

Our measure of whites' perceptions of being on the losing side of health policy was also limited in a few other ways. First, we did not assess other components of relative deprivation that might moderate the effects of loser perceptions (e.g., Crosby 1976): whether respondents felt that they were entitled to better health policies, whether they thought it was feasible to be on the winning side of health policies, and whether they made internal or external attributions for why they were on the losing side. Although, in this context, it is likely that whites who perceived themselves to be on the losing side of health policies felt that they were unjustly so, future research should explicitly measure perceptions of entitlement, feasibility, and attributions of responsibility. Second, to be consistent with the general political loser question, we chose not to include a middle option (i.e., neither winning nor losing). Whereas some research has found no differences in the univariate distribution of responses to a question that includes versus does not include a middle option (Schuman and Presser 1996), other research has found this not to be the case (Bishop 1987). Future research might experiment with using a middle response option to assess the distribution of loser perceptions. Finally, our measure is agnostic as to whether whites who perceive themselves to be on the losing side of health policy view this as a recent (and possibly transient) development, or whether they view it as a more chronic state. Such temporal perceptions could moderate the range, intensity, and direction of the effects on policy attitudes.

Future research also should examine these phenomena in more representative samples and examine the duration of the (admittedly weak) effect of the comparative frame on whites' loser perceptions (see, e.g., Lecheler and de Vreese 2016). It is also important to examine whether frames for the opioid epidemic (e.g., emphasizing white mortality) have different types of effects than do frames for other conditions that exhibit health disparities in outcomes but for the opposite group comparisons, such as diabetes or heart disease.

Table 1 Descriptive Characteristics of Participants in the Control Condition (N = 535)

Characteristic	% or mean
Male	45.4%
Age, year	
Less than 30	29.2%
30–39	36.1%
40–49	15.9%
50+	18.7%
Partisanship	
Republican (includes leaners)	40.6%
Independents	11.4%
Democrats (includes leaners)	48.0%
Ideology (1 = very liberal, 7 = very conservative)	Mean = 3.61
Subjective social status (out of 10)	Mean = 5.32
Household income	
<$27,500	18.9%
$27,500–$49,999	24.7%
$50,000–$74,999	26.2%
$75,000 or more	30.3%
Educational attainment	
High school degree or less	9.7%
Some college	32.8%
Bachelor's	40.6%
More than bachelor's degree	16.9%
Hispanic/Latinx	9.2%
Strength of white identity (out of 7)	Mean = 3.46

Note: The study sample was restricted to respondents who identified their race as white.

Finally, we recognize that a limitation of this study is treating whites as a monolithic group. There are important differences between whites (or within any racial group) in how they view the opioid epidemic based on their relationship to addiction (in self, family, and social networks), their region of residence, and whether they come from an urban or rural environment. In particular, knowing more about respondents' health status, and whether they themselves or close others have experienced addiction would help us better understand the relationships we identified. We are not able to address, for instance, whether those who perceived whites to be on the losing side of health policy had less empathetic responses to the epidemic because they had more intense (and possibly negative) personal experiences with family members or friends with opioid addiction. We also did not have information about rurality of respondents' residence that

Table 2 Predictors of Whites' Perceptions of Being on the Losing Side with Regard to Politics and Health Policy (N = 535)

	Politics loser	Health policy loser
Male	−.05*	−.01
	(.02)	(.02)
Age 30–39 years (compared to <30)	.00	.04
	(.03)	(.03)
Age 40–49 years (compared to <30)	.07+	.10**
	(.04)	(.04)
Age 50 years or older (compared to <30)	.10**	.09**
	(.04)	(.04)
Republican (compared to Democrats)	−.25***	.06+
	(.03)	(.03)
Independents (compared to Democrats)	.00	.12**
	(.04)	(.04)
Ideology (toward conservative)	−.30***	.19***
	(.05)	(.05)
Subjective social status	−.23**	−.24***
	(.07)	(.07)
Income <$27,500 (compared to $75K+)	−.07+	−.01
	(.04)	(.04)
$27,500–$49,999 (compared to $75K+)	−.02	−.02
	(.04)	(.03)
$50,000–$74,999 (compared to $75K+)	.01	.02
	(.03)	(.03)
Hispanic/Latinx	−.08+	.05
	(.04)	(.04)
High school degree or less (compared to BA+)	−.09+	−.00
	(.05)	(.05)
Some college (compared to BA+)	−.09*	−.03
	(.04)	(.04)
Bachelor's (compared to BA+)	−.10**	−.02
	(.04)	(.03)
Strength of white identity	−.09***	−0.02
	(.06)	(0.05)
Constant	1.00***	.27***
	(.07)	(.38)
N	532	533
Adj. R^2	.36	0.11

Notes: The table reports unstandardized regression coefficients from the control group only. Standard errors in parentheses; all variables are scaled to run from 0 to 1.
   + $p < .10$, * $p < .05$, ** $p < .01$, *** $p < .001$.

Table 3 Association of Loser Perceptions on Opioid Policy Attitudes: Empathetic Responses, Punitive Responses, and Stigma

Dependent variable	Perceptions that "your side" is losing in the political domain	Perceptions that whites are losing in the health policy domain	Adj R^2	N
Empathetic attitudes				
Policy scale	.00	−.13***	.24	523
	(.03)	(.03)		
Responsibility: health	.05	−.07+	.06	527
care sector	(.04)	(.04)		
Responsibility: federal	.09*	−.13***	.08	531
government	(.04)	(.04)		
Spending on treatment	.06	−.14***	.16	531
	(.04)	(.04)		
Spending on overdose	.07+	−.14***	.15	531
prevention	(.04)	(.04)		
Spending on education	.08*	−.09*	.10	532
	(.04)	(.04)		
Punitive attitudes				
Policy scale	−.11***	−.01	.27	524
	(.03)	(.03)		
Responsibility: dealers	.15***	−.05	.11	529
	(.05)	(.05)		
Responsibility: users	.03	.08+	.11	531
	(.04)	(.04)		
Responsibility: law	−.05	−.06	.06	529
enforcement	(.04)	(.04)		
Spending on law	.05	.00	.10	528
enforcement: dealers	(.04)	(.04)		
Spending on law	−.04	.01	.14	529
enforcement: users	(.04)	(.04)		
Opioid user feeling	−.07	−.04	.08	531
thermometer	(.04)	(.05)		

Notes: Models adjusted for all characteristics shown in table 2. Each row is a separate regression model. The table reports unstandardized regression coefficients from the control group only. All variables are scaled to run from 0 to 1. Standard errors in parentheses $+ p < 0.10$, $* p < .05$, $** p < .01$, $*** p < .001$

would have been required to better disaggregate white racial identity and its political consequences (see, e.g., Cramer 2016). Future research might also examine whether any framing effects or the relationship between feeling like a loser and policy attitudes might be moderated by the extent to which respondents feel a sense of linked fate (Dawson 1994) with other

Table 4   Effect of Experimental Conditions (Compared to Control Condition) on Loser Perceptions

	Perceptions that "your side" is losing the political domain		Perceptions that whites are losing in the health policy domain	
	(1)	(2)	(1)	(2)
Absolute condition	.02	.02	.02	.02
	(.02)	(.02)	(.02)	(.02)
Comparative condition	.01	−.00	.03+	.04*
	(.02)	(.02)	(.02)	(.02)
With control variables	*No*	*Yes*	*No*	*Yes*
R^2	.00	.38	0.00	.12
N	1547	1537	1545	1536

Note: Unstandardized OLS regression coefficients are reported; numbers in parentheses are standard errors. Control variables for the following characteristics were included: gender, age, partisanship, ideology, subjective social status, income, Hispanic/Latinx ethnicity, education, and strength of white identity.
+ $p < .10$, * $p < .05$

Table 5   Effect of Experimental Conditions (Compared to Control Condition) on Opioid Policy Attitudes

	Empathetic policy scale		Punitive policy scale	
	(1)	(2)	(1)	(2)
Absolute condition	.03**	.04***	−.00	−.00
	(.01)	(.01)	(.01)	(.01)
Comparative condition	.02+	.02	.01	.00
	(.01)	(.01)	(.01)	(.01)
With control variables	*No*	*Yes*	*No*	*Yes*
R^2	.00	.18	.00	.20
N	1523	1513	1521	1511

Note: Unstandardized OLS regression coefficients are reported; numbers in parentheses are standard errors. Control variables for the following characteristics were included: gender, age, partisanship, ideology, subjective social status, income, Hispanic/Latinx ethnicity, education, and strength of white identity.
+ $p < .10$, ** $p < .01$, *** $p < .001$

whites. Schildkraut (2017) finds that linked fate is positively correlated with whites' belief in the importance of having white political candidates, although Gay et al. (2016) find no relationship between linked fate and party identification, ideology, or political participation among a variety of groups, including whites.

Scholars have recently been paying much more attention to examining the connections among health and political behavior, examining, for instance, how community health factors related to the 2016 election (e.g., Bor 2017) or how health insurance gains relate to voter turnout (e.g., Haselswerdt 2017). Whereas these studies at the community or aggregate level are important, our study suggests that future studies at the intersection of health and politics should also engage more deeply at the *individual* level, to consider the underlying political psychological factors that may be politically consequential in how groups determine the appropriate scope of policy in combating public health challenges.

■ ■ ■

Sarah E. Gollust is an associate professor of health policy and management at the University of Minnesota and is an associate director of the Robert Wood Johnson Foundation Interdisciplinary Research Leaders. Her research examines the influence of media and public opinion in the health policy process, the dissemination of research into policy making, and the politics of health policy. Her research has been funded by the National Institutes of Health, the Robert Wood Johnson Foundation, the Russell Sage Foundation, and the American Cancer Society.
sgollust@umn.edu

Joanne M. Miller is an associate professor with a joint appointment in the Department of Political Science and International Relations and the Department of Psychological and Brain Sciences at the University of Delaware. Her research focuses on the psychological and political antecedents of belief in conspiracy theories, the micro and macro causes of political interest, and the motivations for political participation. She has won best paper awards from the following American Political Science Association sections: Elections, Public Opinion, and Voting Behavior; Political Communication; and Political Organizations and Parties; and her research has been funded by the National Science Foundation and the Pew Charitable Trusts.

Acknowledgments

We thank the participants at the Brown University workshop on the Politics of the Opioid Epidemic for their feedback. We also thank the Grand Challenges Research Initiative at the University of Minnesota for funding and Emma Klinger for her research assistance. We received helpful feedback on earlier versions of this article from participants at the American Political Science Association 2018 annual meeting as well as from participants at the Media and Politics Research Group at the University of Minnesota, particularly Benjamin Toff.

References

Adler, Nancy, Elissa S. Epel, Grace Castellazzo, and Jeannette R. Ickovics. 2000. "Relationship of Subjective and Objective Social Status with Psychological and Physiological Functioning: Preliminary Data in Healthy White Women." *Health Psychology* 19, no. 6: 586–92.

Anderson, Christopher J., and Andrew J. LoTempio. 2002. "Winning, Losing, and Political Trust in America." *British Journal of Political Science* 32, no. 2: 335–51.

Armstrong, Elizabeth M., Daniel P. Carpenter, and Marie Hojnacki. 2006. "Whose Deaths Matter? Mortality, Advocacy, and Attention to Disease in the Mass Media." *Journal of Health Politics, Policy and Law* 31, no. 4: 729–72.

Barker, David C., Shaun Bowler, Christopher Jan Carman, and Morten Wendelbo. 2019. "Compromise Is for Losers? Socio-Political Power, Threat, and Public Resistance to Political Compromise." Paper presented at the annual meeting of the American Political Science Association, Washington, DC, August 29–September 1.

Barry, Colleen L., Alene Kennedy-Hendricks, Sarah E. Gollust, Jeff Niederdeppe, Marcus A. Bachhuber, Daniel W. Webster, and Emma E. McGinty. 2016. "Understanding Americans' Views on Opioid Pain Reliever Abuse." *Addiction* 111, no. 1: 85–93.

Benz, Jennifer K., Oscar Espinosa, Valerie Welsh, and Angela Fontes. 2011. "Awareness of Racial and Ethnic Health Disparities Has Improved Only Modestly over a Decade." *Health Affairs* 30, no. 10: 1860–67.

Berinsky, Adam J., Gregory A. Huber, Gabriel S. Lenz, and R. Michael Alvarez. 2012. "Evaluating Online Labor Markets for Experimental Research: Amazon.com's Mechanical Turk." *Political Analysis* 20, no. 3: 351–68.

Best, Rachel Kahn. 2012. "Disease Politics and Medical Research Funding: Three Ways Advocacy Shapes Policy." *American Sociological Review* 77, no. 5: 780–803.

Bigman, Cabral A. 2014. "Social Comparison Framing in Health News and Its Effect on Perceptions of Group Risk." *Health Communication* 29, no. 3: 267–80.

Bishop, George F. 1987. "Experiments with the Middle Response Alternative in Survey Questions." *Public Opinion Quarterly* 51, no. 2: 220–32.

Booske, Bridget C., Stephanie Robert, and Angela M. K. Rohan. 2011. "Awareness of Racial and Socioeconomic Health Disparities in the United States: The National Opinion Survey on Health and Health Disparities, 2008–2009." *Preventing Chronic Disease* 8, no. 4: A73.

Bor, Jacob. 2017. "Diverging Life Expectancies and Voting Patterns in the 2016 US Presidential Election." *American Journal of Public Health* 107, no. 10: 1560–62.

Braveman, Paula A., Shiriki Kumanyika, Jonathan E. Fielding, Thomas Laveist, Luisa N. Borrell, Ron Manderscheid, and Adewale Troutman. 2011. "Health Disparities and Health Equity: The Issue Is Justice." *American Journal of Public Health* 101, suppl. 1: S149–55.

Brown, Lauren, and Reginald Tucker-Seeley. 2018. "Will 'Deaths of Despair' among Whites Change How We Talk about Racial/Ethnic Health Disparities?" *Ethnicity and Disease* 28, no. 2: 123–28.

Buhrmester, Michael, Tracy Kwang, and Samuel D. Gosling. 2011. "Amazon's Mechanical Turk: A New Source of Inexpensive, Yet High-Quality, Data?" *Perspectives on Psychological Science* 6, no. 1: 3–5.

Case, Anne, and Angus Deaton. 2015. "Rising Morbidity and Mortality in Midlife among White Non-Hispanic Americans in the 21st Century." *Proceedings of the National Academy of Sciences* 112, no. 49: 15078–83.

CDC (Centers for Disease Control and Prevention). 2018. "Opioid Overdose." www
.cdc.gov/drugoverdose/index.html (accessed April 8, 2019).

Chokshi, Niraj. 2018. "Trump Voters Driven by Fear of Losing Status, Not Economic Anxiety, Study Finds." *New York Times*, April 24. www.nytimes.com/2018/04/24
/us/politics/trump-economic-anxiety.html.

Cramer, Katherine J. 2016. *The Politics of Resentment: Rural Consciousness in Wisconsin and the Rise of Scott Walker.* Chicago: University of Chicago Press.

Crosby, Faye. 1976. "A Model of Egoistical Relative Deprivation." *Psychological Review* 83, no. 2: 85.

Crump, Matthew J. C., John V. McDonnell, and Todd M. Gureckis. 2013. "Evaluating Amazon's Mechanical Turk as a Tool for Experimental Behavioral Research." *PloS ONE* 8, no. 3: e57410.

Dawson, Michael C. 1994. *Behind the Mule: Race and Class in African-American Politics.* Princeton, NJ: Princeton University Press.

Edelson, Jack, Alexander Alduncin, Christopher Krewson, James A. Sieja, and Joseph E. Uscinski. 2017. "The Effect of Conspiratorial Thinking and Motivated Reasoning on Belief in Election Fraud." *Political Research Quarterly* 70, no. 4: 933–46.

Egan, Jennifer. 2018. "Children of the Opioid Epidemic." *New York Times*, May 9. www.nytimes.com/2018/05/09/magazine/children-of-the-opioid-epidemic.html.

Entman, Robert M. 1993. "Framing: Toward Clarification of a Fractured Paradigm." *Journal of Communication* 43, no. 4: 51–58.

Farhart, Christina. 2017. "Look Who Is Disaffected Now: Political Causes and Consequences of Learned Helplessness in the US." PhD diss., University of Minnesota.

Feldman, Stanley, and Leonie Huddy. 2005. "Racial Resentment and White Opposition to Race-Conscious Programs: Principles or Prejudice?" *American Journal of Political Science* 49, no. 1: 168–83.

Fingerhut, Hannah. 2015. "In Politics, Most Americans Feel They're on the Losing Side." Pew Research Center, November 25. www.pewresearch.org/fact-tank/2015
/11/25/winners-and-losers-in-politics/.

Gay, Claudine, Jennifer Hochschild, and Ariel White. 2016. "Americans' Belief in Linked Fate: Does the Measure Capture the Concept?" *Journal of Race, Ethnicity, and Politics* 1, no. 1: 117–44.

Gollust, Sarah E., and Joseph N. Cappella. 2014. "Understanding Public Resistance to Messages about Health Disparities." *Journal of Health Communication* 19, no. 4: 493–510.

Gollust, Sarah E., and Paula Lantz. 2009. "Communicating Population Health: Print News Media Coverage of Type 2 Diabetes." *Social Science and Medicine* 69, no. 7: 1091–98.

Goodman, Joseph K., Cynthia E. Cryder, and Amar Cheema. 2013. "Data Collection in a Flat World: The Strengths and Weaknesses of Mechanical Turk Samples." *Journal of Behavioral Decision Making* 26, no. 3: 213–24.

Goodwin, James S., Yong-Fang Kuo, David Brown, David Juurlink, and Mukaila Raji. 2018. "Association of Chronic Opioid Use with Presidential Voting Patterns in US Counties in 2016." *JAMA Network Open* 1, no. 2: e180450.

Gurney, Joan Neff, and Kathleen J. Tierney. 1982. "Relative Deprivation and Social Movements: A Critical Look at Twenty Years of Theory and Research." *Sociological Quarterly* 23, no. 1: 33–47.

Hansen, Helena, and Julie Netherland. 2016. "Is the Prescription Opioid Epidemic a White Problem?" *American Journal of Public Health* 106, no. 12: 2127–29.

Harbin, M. Brielle. 2019. "The Contingency of Compassion: Media Depictions of Drug Addiction." Unpublished paper.

Haselswerdt, Jake. 2017. "Expanding Medicaid, Expanding the Electorate: The Affordable Care Act's Short-Term Impact on Political Participation." *Journal of Health Politics, Policy and Law* 42, no. 4: 667–95.

Jamison, Peter. 2018. "Falling Out: A Generation of African American Heroin Users Is Dying in the Opioid Epidemic Nobody Talks About. The Nation's Capital Is Ground Zero." *Washington Post*, December 18. www.washingtonpost.com/graphics/2018/local/opioid-epidemic-and-its-effects-on-african-americans.

Jardina, Ashley. 2019. *White Identity Politics*. Cambridge: Cambridge University Press.

Kennedy-Hendricks, Alene, Colleen L. Barry, Sarah E. Gollust, Margaret E. Ensminger, Margaret S. Chisolm, and Emma E. McGinty. 2017. "Social Stigma toward Persons with Prescription Opioid Use Disorder: Associations with Public Support for Punitive and Public Health–Oriented Policies." *Psychiatric Services* 68, no. 5: 462–69.

KFF (Kaiser Family Foundation). n.d. "Opioid Overdose Deaths by Race/Ethnicity." State Health Facts. kff.org/other/state-indicator/opioid-overdose-deaths-by-raceethnicity/ (accessed November 12, 2019).

Kinder, Donald, and Lynn Sanders. 1996. *Divided by Color: Racial Politics and Democratic Ideals*. Chicago: University of Chicago Press.

Lecheler, Sophie, and Claus H. de Vreese. 2016. "How Long Do News Framing Effects Last? A Systematic Review of Longitudinal Studies." *Annals of the International Communication Association* 40, no. 1: 3–30.

Levay, Kevin E., Jeremy Freese, and James N. Druckman. 2016. "The Demographic and Political Composition of Mechanical Turk Samples." *Sage Open* January-March: 1–17. doi.org/10.1177/2158244016636433.

Lopez, German. 2017. "When a Drug Epidemic's Victims Are White." *Vox*, April 4. www.vox.com/identities/2017/4/4/15098746/opioid-heroin-epidemic-race.

Luhtanen, Riia, and Jennifer Crocker. 1992. "A Collective Self-Esteem Scale: Self-Evaluation of One's Social Identity." *Personality and Social Psychology Bulletin* 18, no. 3: 302–18.

Lynch, Julia, and Sarah E. Gollust. 2010. "Playing Fair: Fairness Beliefs and Health Policy Preferences in the United States." *Journal of Health Politics Policy Law* 35, no. 6: 849–87.

MacKinnon, David P., and Angela G. Pirlott. 2015. "Statistical Approaches for Enhancing Causal Interpretation of the M to Y Relation in Mediation Analysis." *Personality and Social Psychology Review* 19, no. 1: 30–43.

McGinty, Emma Beth., Alene Kennedy-Hendricks, Julia Baller, Jeff Niederdeppe, Sarah Gollust, and Colleen L. Barry. 2016. "Criminal Activity or Treatable Health Condition? News Media Framing of Opioid Analgesic Abuse in the United States, 1998–2012." *Psychiatric Services* 67, no. 4: 405–11.

McGinty, Emma E., Colleen L. Barry, Elizabeth M. Stone, Jeff Niederdeppe, Alene Kennedy-Hendricks, Sarah Linden, and Susan G. Sherman. 2018. "Public Support for Safe Consumption Sites and Syringe Services Programs to Combat the Opioid Epidemic." *Preventive Medicine* 111: 73–77.

Metzl, Jonathan. 2019. *Dying of Whiteness: How the Politics of Racial Resentment Is Killing America's Heartland.* New York: Basic Books.

Miller, Joanne M., Kyle Saunders, and Christina Farhart. 2018. "The Relationship between Losing an Election and Conspiracy Theory Endorsement." Paper presented at the annual conference of the Midwest Political Science Association, Chicago, IL, April 5–9.

Monnat, Shannon M., and David L. Brown. 2017. "More than a Rural Revolt: Landscapes of Despair and the 2016 Presidential Election." *Journal of Rural Studies* 55: 227–36.

Nadeau, Richard, and André Blais. 1993. "Accepting the Election Outcome: The Effect of Participation on Losers' Consent." *British Journal of Political Science* 23, no. 4: 553–63.

Nagler, Rebekah H., Cabral A. Bigman, Shoba Ramanadhan, Divya Ramamurthi, and K. Viswanath. 2016. "Prevalence and Framing of Health Disparities in Local Print News: Implications for Multilevel Interventions to Address Cancer Inequalities." *Cancer Epidemiology Biomarkers and Prevention* 25, no. 4: 603–12.

Netherland, Julie, and Helena B. Hansen. 2016. "The War on Drugs That Wasn't: Wasted Whiteness, 'Dirty Doctors,' and Race in Media Coverage of Prescription Opioid Misuse." *Culture, Medicine, and Psychiatry* 40, no. 4: 664–86.

Nicholson, Robert A., Matthew W. Kreuter, Christina Lapka, Rachel Wellborn, Eddie M. Clark, Vetta Sanders-Thompson, Heather M. Jacobsen, and Chris Casey. 2008. "Unintended Effects of Emphasizing Disparities in Cancer Communication to African-Americans." *Cancer Epidemiology, Biomarkers, and Prevention* 17, no. 11: 2946–53.

Niederdeppe, Jeff, Cabral A. Bigman, Amy L. Gonzales, and Sarah E. Gollust. 2013. "Communication about Health Disparities in the Mass Media." *Journal of Communication* 63, no. 1: 8–30.

Pettigrew, Thomas F. 2015. "Samuel Stouffer and Relative Deprivation." *Social Psychology Quarterly* 78, no. 1: 7–24.

Pew Research Center. 2018. "Key Findings on Americans' Views of the US Political System and Democracy." Fact Tank, April 26. www.pewresearch.org/fact-tank/2018/04/26/key-findings-on-americans-views-of-the-u-s-political-system-and-democracy/.

Rothman, Alexander J., Roger D. Bartels, Jhon Wlaschin, and Peter Salovey. 2006. "The Strategic Use of Gain- and Loss-Framed Messages to Promote Healthy Behavior: How Theory Can Inform Practice." *Journal of Communication* 56, suppl. 1: S202–20.

Runciman, Walter Garrison. 1993. *Relative Deprivation and Social Justice: A Study of Attitudes to Social Inequality in Twentieth-Century England.* Berkeley: University of California Press.

Saloner, Brendon, and Colleen L. Barry. 2018. "Ending the Opioid Epidemic Requires a Historic Investment in Medication-Assisted Treatment." *Journal of Policy Analysis and Management* 37, no. 2: 431–38.

Schildkraut, Deborah J. 2017. "White Attitudes about Descriptive Representation in the US: The Roles of Identity, Discrimination, and Linked Fate." *Politics, Groups, and Identities* 5, no. 1: 84–106.

Schuman, Howard, and Stanley Presser. 1996. *Questions and Answers in Attitude Surveys: Experiments on Question Form, Wording, and Context.* Thousand Oaks, CA: Sage.

Smith, Heather J., and Yuen J. Huo. 2014. "Relative Deprivation: How Subjective Experiences of Inequality Influence Social Behavior and Health." *Policy Insights from the Behavioral and Brain Sciences* 1, no. 1: 231–38.

Sweeney, Paul D., Dean B. McFarlin, and Edward J. Inderrieden. 1990. "Using Relative Deprivation Theory to Explain Satisfaction with Income and Pay Level: A Multistudy Examination." *Academy of Management Journal* 33, no. 2: 423–36.

Subramanyam, Malavika, Ichiro Kawachi, Lisa Berkman, and S. V. Subramanian. 2009. "Relative Deprivation in Income and Self-Rated Health in the United States." *Social Science and Medicine* 69, no. 3: 327–34.

Wasfy, Jason H., Charles Stewart III, and Vijeta Bhambhani. 2017. "County Community Health Associations of Net Voting Shift in the 2016 US Presidential Election." *PloS ONE* 12, no. 10: e0185051.

Weinberg, Jill D., Jeremy Freese, and David McElhattan. 2014. "Comparing Data Characteristics and Results of an Online Factorial Survey between a Population-Based and a Crowdsource-Recruited Sample." *Sociological Science*, August 4. www.sociologicalscience.com/articles-vol1-19-292/.

Weiner, Bernard. 2006. *Social Motivation, Justice, and the Moral Emotions: An Attributional Approach.* Mahwah, NJ: Lawrence Erlbaum Associates.

Appendix 1: Treatment Articles

Absolute Frame Article

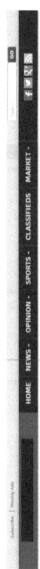

Rising Opioid Addictions Pose a Threat to Health of White Americans

By Melissa Paulhus

Washington, DC. A conference about opioid addiction that was organized by Trust for America's Health, a non-profit, non-partisan public health organization, convened here this week. People addicted to opioids abuse prescription drugs like morphine or oxycodone or illegal drugs like heroin. The addiction can cause serious health complications, including death. White Americans have been hit particularly hard by this public health threat, according to new data released at the conference. The rate of opioid overdose deaths among whites is 17.5 per 100,000; this amounts to 33,450 total deaths among whites in 2016.

The conference, held June 22-24, brought scientists, doctors, drug manufacturers, insurers, and affected patients and family members together to discuss the rising rates of overdose from opioids, including prescription pain medications and illegal drugs like heroin, that have plagued white communities in states across the nation in recent years. Dr. Eugene Smith, one of the speakers at the conference said, "The medical community is still searching for the reasons why this health challenge has been so deeply felt among whites."

The rate of drug overdoses nationally has tripled since 1999. In Ohio, the drug overdose rate among whites is 37.0 per 100,000

(which is twice the national average) and 3,217 white people died of opioid overdoses in that state in 2016, according to data released at the meeting.

Treating opioid addiction and responding to emergency overdoses is one part of the solution, said conference presenters. However, the real challenge is figuring out the best way to prevent opioid addiction in the first place. The next phase of the conference – to be convened later in the fall – will focus on developing recommendations for prevention.

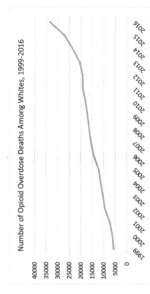

Number of Opioid Overdose Deaths Among Whites, 1999-2016

Comparative Frame Article

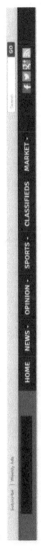

Rising Opioid Addictions Pose a Greater Threat to Health of White Americans than Black Americans

By Melissa Paulhus

Washington, DC. A conference about opioid addiction that was organized by Trust for America's Health, a non-profit, non-partisan public health organization, convened here this week. People addicted to opioids abuse prescription drugs like morphine or oxycodone or illegal drugs like heroin. The addiction can cause serious health complications, including death. White Americans have been hit particularly hard by this public health threat compared to black Americans, according to new data released at the conference. The rate of drug overdose deaths among whites is 17.5 per 100,000 compared to 10.3 among blacks; this amounts to 33,450 total deaths among whites and 4,374 deaths among blacks in 2016.

The conference, held June 22-24, brought scientists, doctors, drug manufacturers, insurers, and affected patients and family members together to discuss the rising rates of overdose from opioids, including prescription pain medications and illegal drugs like heroin, that have plagued white communities in states across the nation in recent years. Predominantly black communities have not experienced rising rates of overdose. Dr. Eugene Smith, one of the speakers at the conference said, "The medical community is still searching for the reasons why this health challenge has been so deeply felt among whites but less so among blacks."

The rate of drug overdoses nationally has tripled since 1999. In Ohio, the drug overdose rate among whites is 37.0 per 100,000

(which is twice the national average) and 3,217 whites died of opioid overdoses in that state in 2016, compared to 322 deaths among blacks, according to data released at the meeting.

Treating opioid addiction and responding to emergency overdoses is one part of the solution, said conference presenters. However, the real challenge is figuring out the best way to prevent opioid addiction in the first place. The next phase of the conference – to be convened later in the fall – will focus on developing recommendations for prevention.

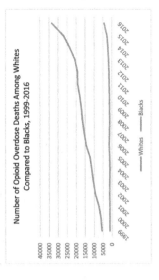

Number of Opioid Overdose Deaths Among Whites Compared to Blacks, 1999-2016

Appendix 2: Support for Policies to Address the Opioid Epidemic, Control Group Only

How much do you favor or oppose the following policy to address the problem of opioid (prescription pain medication and heroin) abuse? (7-point scale, higher values = more favorability)

Policy	Control group mean
Policies we classified as empathetic	
Requiring insurance companies to provide coverage for treatment of substance abuse problems.	5.27
Providing friends and family members of people using opioids with access to naloxone (also known as Narcan), which is a medication that can quickly and effectively help a person experiencing a drug overdose.	5.06
Passing laws to protect people from criminal charges for drug crimes if they seek help for themselves or others experiencing an opioid overdose.	5.10
Developing health education campaigns to reduce the stigma the public holds toward those who use opioids.	5.10
Expanding availability of drug testing kits so that people who use opioids can test the drugs for lethal substances such as fentanyl.	4.76
Increase availability of health care providers who prescribe medication-assisted treatment (e.g., methadone, buprenorphine).	5.14
Policies we classified as punitive	
Arresting and prosecuting people who are in possession of opioids.	4.42
Arresting and prosecuting drug dealers and drug traffickers.	5.81
Restricting immigration from countries such as Mexico that are involved in the illegal drug trade.	4.22
Arresting and prosecuting health care providers who prescribe opioids without following existing regulations.	5.42
Arresting and prosecuting parents who are addicted to opioids on criminal child abuse charges.	4.55
Requiring health care providers to report women who have abused opioids during pregnancy to child welfare authorities.	5.19

Appendix 3: Question Wording and Coding for Control Variables

Party identification. Respondents were first asked, "Generally speaking, do you usually think of yourself as a Democrat, a Republican, an Independent, or what?" Respondents who responded Democrat or Republican were then asked, "Would you call yourself a strong Democrat [Republican] or a not very strong Democrat [Republican]?" Respondents who responded Independent or other were then asked, "Do you think of yourself as closer to the Democratic Party or the Republican Party?" (with "neither" included as a response option). Responses were coded as two dummy variables representing Republicans/Republican leaners and Democrats/Democratic leaners, with pure Independents as the comparison group.

Ideology. Respondents were asked, "We hear a lot of talk these days about liberals and conservatives. Here is a 7-point scale on which the political views that people might hold are arranged from extremely liberal to extremely conservative. Where would you place yourself on this scale?" The 7-point scale was coded to range from 0–1; higher numbers = more conservative.

Gender. Respondents' self-reported gender was coded such that 1 = male and 0 = female.

Income. We assessed income with the following question: "The next question is about the total income of YOUR HOUSEHOLD for the PAST 12 MONTHS. Please include your income PLUS the income of all members living in your household (including cohabiting partners and armed forces members living at home). Please count income BEFORE TAXES, including income from all sources (such as wages, salaries, tips, net income from a business, interest, dividends, child support, alimony, Social Security, public assistance, pensions, and retirement benefits)." Respondents were asked to choose 1 of 28 income groupings, which were then recoded into 3 dummy variables: less than or equal to $27,599; $27,500–$49,999; and $50,000–$74,999, with $75,000 and up as the comparison group.

Age. Respondents' reported age was coded into three dummy variables: 30–39 years; 40–49 years; and 50 years or older, with younger than 30 years as the comparison group.

Education. Respondents were asked, "What is the highest level of school you have completed or the highest degree you have received?" They were given 10 categories from which to choose. Responses were recoded into three dummy variables: high school or less; some college; and bachelor's degree, with more than a bachelor's degree serving as the comparison group.

Latinx ethnicity. Respondents were asked, "Are you Spanish, Hispanic, or Latino?" (coded such that 1 = Hispanic/Latinx identity and 0 = not Hispanic/Latinx identity).

Strength of white identity. Strength of white identity was assessed with four items developed by Luhtanen and Crocker 1992 (each measured on a 7-point agree-disagree Likert scale): "Being White has very little to do with how I feel about myself" (reverse-coded), "Being White is an important reflection of who I am", "Being White is unimportant to my sense of what kind of person I am" (reverse-coded), and "Being White is an important part of my self-image." Responses were recoded to range from 0–1 and then averaged to form an index.

Subjective perception of relative socioeconomic status. We used the MacArthur Scale of Subjective Social Status, Adult Version (see Adler et al. 2000), to assess subjective perceptions of socioeconomic status. Respondents were shown a picture of a ladder with 10 rungs numbered 1–10 and were given the following instructions (responses were coded to range from 0–1):

> **"Think of this ladder as representing where people stand in the United States.** At the **top** of the ladder are the people who are the best off—those who have the most money, the most education, and the most respected jobs. At the **bottom** are the people who are the worst off—those who have the least money, least education, and the least respected jobs or no job. The higher up you are on this ladder, the closer you are to the people at the very top; the lower you are, the closer you are to the people at the very bottom. **Where would you place yourself on this ladder?** Please type the whole number that represents the rung where you think you stand at this time in your life, relative to other people in the United States."

Are Policy Strategies for Addressing the Opioid Epidemic Partisan? A View from the States

Colleen M. Grogan
University of Chicago

Clifford S. Bersamira
University of Hawaiʻi

Phillip M. Singer
University of Utah

Bikki Tran Smith
Harold A. Pollack
University of Chicago

Christina M. Andrews
University of South Carolina

Amanda J. Abraham
University of Georgia

Abstract
Context: In contrast to the Affordable Care Act, some have suggested the opioid epidemic represents an area of bipartisanship. This raises an important question: to what extent are Democrat-led and Republican-led states different or similar in their policy responses to the opioid epidemic?
Methods: Three main methodological approaches were used to assess state-level policy responses to the opioid epidemic: a legislative analysis across all 50 states, an online survey of 50 state Medicaid agencies, and in-depth case studies with policy stakeholders in five states.
Findings: Conservative states pursue hidden and targeted Medicaid expansions, and a number of legislative initiatives, to address the opioid crisis. However, the total fiscal commitment among these Republican-led states pales in comparison to states that adopt the ACA Medicaid expansion. Because the state legislative initiatives do not provide treatment, these states spend substantially less than states with Democratic control.
Conclusions: Rather than persistently working to retrench all programs, conservatives have relied on policy designs that emphasize devolution, fragmentation, and inequality to both expand and retrench benefits. This strategy, which allocates benefits differentially to different social groups and obfuscates responsibility, allows conservatives to avoid political blame typically associated with retrenchment.

Keywords   opioid politics, Medicaid, retrenchment

Journal of Health Politics, Policy and Law, Vol. 45, No. 2, April 2020
DOI 10.1215/03616878-8004886   © 2020 by Duke University Press

One of the most notable political aspects of the Affordable Care Act (ACA) is the extreme partisanship that accompanied both its enactment and the postenactment period. Not one Republican voted for the ACA, and their high level of opposition to the bill was sustained from when it was passed in 2010 through 2017 (Hacker and Pierson 2018; Patashnik and Oberlander 2018). Immediately after the bill passed, 23 Republican-led states joined a lawsuit challenging the individual mandate and claiming that the Medicaid expansion represented federal coercion and unduly restricted states' rights. While the Supreme Court upheld the individual mandate, it ruled in favor of the states' claim about Medicaid. As a result, the federal government could allow states to adopt the Medicaid expansion but not mandate it (Grogan 2014; Rosenbaum 2012; see also Grogan and Jacobson 2013). States' embrace or rejection of the Medicaid expansion exemplified the political polarization around the ACA. Initially, all of the Democrat-led states adopted the Medicaid expansion, and almost all Republican-led states refused it.

At the same time, the opioid epidemic was growing in nearly every state across the country. Opioid overdose deaths quadrupled from 1999 to 2015 and accounted for almost all of the increase in overdose deaths over the past decade (O'Donnell, Gladden and Seth 2017; Rudd et al. 2016; Scholl et al. 2018). The societal and economic costs also continued to grow: from 2001 to 2017, the opioid epidemic cost more than $1 trillion, including costs related to lost productivity, tax revenue, health care, social services, education, and criminal justice (Altarum 2018; Segel et al. 2019). Opioid overdose deaths outnumber automobile fatalities nationally, and substantially exceed the annual death toll from AIDS at the peak of the HIV/AIDS epidemic.

Given the overwhelming impact of the opioid epidemic, it is not surprising that the US public believes the government should act to address it. Over two-thirds (69%) of the public believe opioid misuse is a serious (47%) or somewhat serious (22%) problem in their state (Politico/Harvard School of Public Health Poll, July 2018). While Republicans and Democrats both report concern about the problem, there are some partisan differences in beliefs about whether government should respond and how. When asked which entity should have the greatest responsibility for regulating addiction treatment, the vast majority (77%) said government. Yet, when asked whether spending should be increased for the *federal* government to deal with the opioid epidemic, 52% of Democrats supported more spending, compared with only 38% of Republicans and 30% of Independents (Johnson 2017). Most Republicans favor state government action over federal, with 44% believing it should be state government.

However, the severity of the opioid epidemic appears to influence public opinion regarding the role of federal government in responding to it. Fully 55% of respondents who live in states with opioid-related mortality rates exceeding 20 per 100,000 persons support more federal spending on the crisis (Johnson 2017). This is an important distinction because many states with Republican Party control have higher per capita opioid death rates (Goodwin et al. 2018). While some Republican constituencies may not want the federal government to act, the majority — especially in high-need states — want state government action to curb the opioid epidemic.

It is also clear that politicians are feeling pressure to respond to this issue. During the 2018 campaigns, politicians in competitive races used emotional pleas about opioid use disorder (OUD) and misuse to woo voters. In states like Wisconsin, where hundreds of people are dying of opioid overdoses every year, candidates from both parties were talking about drugs in stump speeches, on Facebook, and in ads using startlingly similar language. Some suggest the opioid epidemic represents an area of bipartisanship where members of both parties have found broad areas of agreement (Smith 2018).

This raises an important question, which we seek to address in this article: to what extent are Democrat-led and Republican-led states different or similar in their policy responses to the opioid epidemic? To address this question, we use three data sources: in-depth interviews with stakeholders in five Republican-led states, a survey of 50 state Medicaid agencies to document substance use disorder coverage policy, and proposed and enacted legislation to address the opioid epidemic from 50 state legislatures. Our findings suggest that Republican-led states are indeed feeling significant pressure to respond to the opioid epidemic, and are in some cases taking significant steps to address it. Three of our five case study states indicate that the epidemic was a major driving force that led their states to adopt the Medicaid expansion. Because the Medicaid expansion was completely off the table in two of our case study states, while demand for state action to address the opioid epidemic was similarly intense, these states pursued less-prominent and more-targeted policy approaches in their regular Medicaid programs, and a number of state-level legislative initiatives. Our 50-state survey data corroborated that Republican-led states rely on Medicaid to provide benefits for substance use disorder (SUD). States with total Republican control also passed more legislation to address the opioid epidemic and devoted a higher proportion of state resources to these legislative initiatives than Democrat-led states.

Nonetheless, the total fiscal commitment to address the opioid epidemic among these Republican-led states pales in comparison to states that adopted the Medicaid expansion. Because non-expansion legislative initiatives tend to focus on regulation or raising awareness, these Republican-led actions are more modest than those implemented by states with Democratic control. Because Republicans have not come up with a non-Medicaid policy to expand treatment to address the epidemic, they overall spend substantially less, and leave thousands of people with OUD without access to treatment in their state. Given this reality, it is logical to ask, How can Republicans in these states pursue a policy that denies access to treatment for a core part of their base without political consequences?

Partisanship, Retrenchment, and the Opioid Epidemic

Political polarization in the US has recently been described as asymmetrical because the Republican Party has moved further to the right over time, while Democrats have remained ideologically in place (Bonica 2013; Hacker and Pierson 2015, 2018; Mann and Ornstein 2013; Skocpol and Jacobs 2011). As Jacob S. Hacker and Paul Pierson (2018: 560) note, this movement to the right "can be seen in roll-call votes in Congress, in the positions of presidents and vice presidents, [and] in ideological divisions on the Supreme Court." Under asymmetrical polarization, Republicans have been more willing to pursue retrenchment policies even when their own voter base is against it, such as with their most recent attempt to repeal the ACA in 2017. Indeed, as Republicans were attempting to repeal the ACA, one of the key arguments against it—even among members in their own party—was the impact repeal would have on the opioid epidemic. As Medicaid has expanded over time, even in conservative states, and the Republican Party's core constituents include working-class voters, who ironically rely on the program for a vital source of financial protection and access to care, a sizable portion of their base was against repeal and the significant cuts proposed to Medicaid (Grogan and Park 2018; Hacker and Pierson 2018). Why were Republicans in Washington seemingly unconcerned about a potential backlash among their base?

Hacker and Pierson (2018) offer three reasons. First, in 2017, Republicans had a majority in the House and Senate, and believed this gave them a substantial electoral cushion. Second, Republicans appealed negative partisanship strategies to encourage their base to be driven more by distrust or fear of the other party than by love of their policies. And finally, "Republicans designed their health care bills in ways that aimed to minimize the degree to which voters might mobilize against them. Particularly important was their reliance on the devolution of policy responsibility to the states; . . . strategic policy engineering was meant to provide 'backlash insurance' . . . [to] insulate the party from significant electoral fallout" (562–63).

Yet, if Republican-controlled states focus on retrenchment, how do they avoid political costs associated with cutting popular programs? We argue that the structure of the program allows Republicans to strategically use the program to achieve their own policy objectives while avoiding blame. Because Medicaid is entrenched as a devolved, fragmented, and unequal program, federal-level Republicans fight to continue to keep the program as a devolved, fragmented, and unequal program, while state-level Republicans' oppositional strategy includes targeted retrenchment *and expansion.* While Democrats attempt to entrench a *liberal* version of the welfare state, Republicans pursue strategies to not only resist liberal policies but also embrace a conservative version of the welfare state.

This insight helps explain how conservative policy makers believed they could run a retrenchment, antigovernment campaign at the federal level seemingly without electoral costs, because they can use conservatively designed programs at the state-level such as Medicaid that are devolved, fragmented, and unequal to strategically expand and retract. In addition to employing a negative partisanship frame, we argue that Republicans also use discourse that aligns with their conservative policy designs—devolution, fragmentation, and inequity—to frame expansions targeted to their base as deserving, and retrenchments targeted to those who oppose them as undeserving.

The politics surrounding the opioid epidemic reveals the conservative welfare state strategy in action. When Congress passed the Comprehensive Addiction and Recovery Act (CARA) and 21st Century Cures Act in 2016 and the Substance Use–Disorder Prevention that Promotes Opioid Recovery and Treatment for Patients and Communities (SUPPORT) Act in 2018, it allowed states to reject the Medicaid expansion to solve the opioid crisis and instead (ironically given their stance of accepting federal funding) to draw down federal funds to specifically target the opioid epidemic. CARA authorized many harm-reduction strategies, including increased access to the opioid overdose reversal drug, naloxone. The 21st Century Cures Act designated $1 billion in grants for states over two years to fight the opioid epidemic. The money could be used to make SUD treatment programs more accessible, to improve the quality of the SUD workforce, and to research the most effective approaches to prevent addiction.

The SUPPORT Act offers a range of strategies for addressing the epidemic, including targeting improvements in Medicaid and Medicare programs, expanding access to opioid and nonopioid treatment options and provider capacity,[1] improving oversight of opioid prescribing through increased data sharing, removing barriers to maintenance of coverage for special populations (e.g., pregnant women, infants, and children), expanding use of telehealth, and incorporating housing and other recovery support services in SUD treatment. These programs allow Republicans at the federal level to attempt to avoid blame aimed at Medicaid retrenchment by pointing to these targeted solutions to problems their base cares deeply about. They also allow Republicans to devolve responsibility to the states. We turn now to our methods and then findings to show how states pursue a targeted strategy of expansion and retrenchment to respond to their base and avoid blame for not doing more.

Methods

Three main methodological approaches were used to assess state-level policy responses to the opioid epidemic: a legislative analysis across all 50 states, an online survey of 50 state Medicaid agencies, and in-depth case studies with policy stakeholders in 5 states. Because the Republican Party platform and the majority of Republican constituents explicitly indicated they do not approve of federal action to address the opioid epidemic, but do favor state action, we used states as the unit of analysis, instead of parties or legislators, to see if Republican-led states are indeed acting to address the opioid crisis and, if so, how?

National Analysis of Legislative Action

To understand legislative action across all states, we created a unique dataset of all introduced state legislation related to opioids and the opioid epidemic. The database was created from keyword searches related to the opioid epidemic through LexisNexis databases on state legislation from 2014 through 2018. All legislation was initially scanned to determine if it was related to the opioid epidemic, with unrelated bills excluded from the remainder of the analysis. From the remaining bills that were introduced, the following data was collected: state, year of introduction, whether the legislation was enacted, the legislation sponsor's political party affiliation, the partisan breakdown of floor votes from each chamber, and the type of legislation (regulation, education/public awareness, or treatment).

---

1. As an example of nonopioid treatment options, methadone will become a covered benefit under Medicare Part D beginning in January of 2020.

The coding of this information involved two researchers. To develop the coding scheme of the intention of the legislation, a subset of opioid legislation was selected across different years and states. Using open coding techniques, two researchers read through 100 pieces of legislation and devised an initial coding scheme to catalog the type of legislation. After the coding scheme was developed, the two researchers independently read through an additional 200 pieces of legislation and compared their results. The coders agreed on 85% of the coding, with the remaining discrepancies discussed and adjudicated, adding additional detail to the codebook as well as four additional codes. A single researcher then finished coding the remaining legislation.

Survey of Medicaid Benefit Coverage Policies

To gather data on state Medicaid coverage of SUD treatments that could be used to address the opioid crisis, we conducted a 15-minute, internet-based survey of Medicaid programs in the 50 states. The University of Chicago Survey Lab conducted the survey from May to December in 2017. State Medicaid directors were mailed a packet that contained a description of the study, an invitation to participate, and a request to designate a knowledgeable staff person to fill out the survey. To encourage participation, the survey lab followed up by phone and email with directors who did not respond. Forty-seven Medicaid programs responded, for a 94% response rate. For the three states that did not complete the survey, a research team member added data from an earlier 2014 wave of the survey and verified these data from a review of publicly available resources on state Medicaid coverage for addiction treatment. As a result, the final study data included the total population of the Medicaid programs in all 50 states. Medication data were collected through a review of published state drug formularies using the method employed by the American Society of Addiction Medicine to collect data in 2014.

State Case Studies

To provide more granular analysis, case studies were conducted in five states. Using purposive sampling, state selection was based on four criteria. First, we identified states with high salience of drug and alcohol issues, as measured by national media and state political attention (17 states). We drew from four national newspapers with high readership—the *New York Times*, the *Washington Post*, *USA Today*, and the *Wall Street Journal*. We identified national-level articles' coverage of state-specific prescription-opioid, heroin, alcohol, and other drug issues from 2013 to 2014. Next, governors' State of the State addresses were reviewed for explicit mention of the opioid epidemic (22 states). In states with incoming governors, Inaugural Addresses were reviewed in lieu of State of the State addresses. States were ranked based on the extent of media attention garnered and political attention on substance use issues. States with higher salience were more likely to be chosen as a case site.

Second, we identified states based on whether or not a state had expanded Medicaid. We wanted to ensure that at least half of our sample states had chosen to expand their Medicaid program and include ones that expanded at different times. Third, we wanted to have a mix of states that established their own state health insurance exchanges and states that opted to use the federally facilitated platform. Fourth, to ensure geographic variation, we selected states to include all regions in the United States.

Because this study is particularly interested in shedding light on how Republican-led states have responded to the opioid epidemic, we focus on data from five of the eight states selected that at the time of our study represented total Republican Party control (Ohio, Florida, and Georgia) or ideologically conservative states with divided party control (Kentucky and New Hampshire).

Stakeholder Selection

To capture a comprehensive understanding of states' responses to the opioid epidemic and health policy reform, our recruitment strategy targeted a range of stakeholders in each state using a nonprobabilistic snowball sampling approach to understand the perspectives of diverse political actors (Weiss 1995). Expert interviews targeted stakeholders directly involved in the policy-making process to better understand goal conflicts and technical disputes and to account for the role of multiple actors within the policy community (Sabatier and Weible 2007).

In-depth interviews were conducted via telephone and audio-recorded, with each interview lasting approximately one hour (ranging from 40 to 75 minutes). All interviews were conducted by the study team lead interviewer, accompanied by co-investigators designated by state. Prior to the start of each interview, verbal informed consent was obtained from each participant.

We use the qualitative data to first show how the opioid epidemic was a crucial driver pushing three of our states to adopt the Medicaid expansion, and, second, to shed light on our 50-state Medicaid survey data and state legislative data.

Findings: Front-Stage Retrenchment Politics with Exceptions: The Opioid Epidemic and the Medicaid Expansion

The most notable difference in *how* states address the opioid epidemic relates to whether states adopt the ACA Medicaid expansion. Strong evidence shows that partisan politics plays a large role in explaining which states adopt the Medicaid expansion, with Democrat-controlled states adopting and Republican-controlled states opting out (Barrilleaux and Rainey 2014; Grogan and Park 2017; Lanford and Quadagno 2016). As of 2017, when we conducted the interviews, 32 states including the District of Columbia had adopted the Medicaid expansion (KFF n.d.). Of the 19 states that opted out, 16 were under total Republican control and the remaining 3 were under mixed control.

Although partisanship is the main driver in determining which states adopt the expansion, there were some exceptions: 9 states under total Republican control and 16 states under mixed control adopted the expansion.

Scholars have written about the politics in several conservative states leading to passage of the Medicaid expansion (Grogan, Singer, and Jones 2017; Kliff 2016, 2017), but none have mentioned the role of the opioid epidemic in nudging states toward Medicaid expansion. Our qualitative data suggests that the crisis played an important role in moving three of our five states toward adopting the Medicaid expansion. For example, Ohio is a Republican controlled state, but passed the Medicaid expansion. Mixed party control existed in Kentucky and New Hampshire when these states passed the Medicaid expansion, but in 2016 both switched to total Republican control. Ohio, New Hampshire, and Kentucky rank second, third, and seventh, respectively, in opioid mortality.

All the stakeholders in these states emphasized the personal nature of the opioid epidemic and the direct impact of overdose deaths on the families and local communities of policy makers who are making key health policy decisions. In Kentucky, a state agency representative mentioned that because 1 in 3 "Kentuckians say they know somebody with a substance use disorder," it means that for a lot more people the issue has "a human face" and is personal (KY stakeholder no. 6). In New Hampshire, a Managed Care Organization (MCO) representative noted the pressure put on the state legislature by "a large vocal group of leaders and stakeholders" who demanded "a robust response to the opioid epidemic" (NH stakeholder no. 8). An Ohio state agency representative mentioned how important it was that the political pressure "crossed all socioeconomic layers, [and] brought people to the table" that normally didn't talk to one another. This same representative mentioned that this was a huge shift from just a few years prior, when there was "virtually no investment in this area" (OH stakeholder no. 1).

The urgent nature of the opioid epidemic also fostered a shift in ideological views on how SUD should be addressed. A provider representative in Kentucky said that in the past most thought, "You're a bad person if you're addicted." Because of this mindset, the state supported a punitive approach. However, today, the view is dramatically different with many conservative legislators supporting harm reduction practices. "We went from over a 10-year [stigmatizing] period, to passing legislation that included needle exchange" and a much broader "acceptance of medication-assisted treatment" (KY stakeholder no. 3). An Ohio MCO representative noted that "the vast majority of folks [now view] substance abuse as an illness" as opposed to a behavioral problem, and believe it should "be treated medically" (OH stakeholder no. 2).

Perhaps surprisingly, stakeholders in these Republican-led states discussed how it was viewed as irresponsible *not* to adopt the Medicaid expansion in light of the severity of the epidemic. Because "people are dying" and Medicaid is "one, if not the biggest funders for treating that issue, we can't afford frankly to not pay for services that work for people" (OH stakeholder no. 5, state agency representative). Some noted that the seriousness of the opioid epidemic pushed even some of the most conservative legislators toward accepting the Medicaid expansion. An MCO representative said, "The guys in Ohio . . . that frankly ran and won, on the very, very right side of John Boehner, still support substance abuse and opioid treatment" (OH stakeholder no. 2). They primarily wanted to support treatment for OUD, but realized that the Medicaid expansion was the easiest way to do that.

Although these conservative states were pushed to adopt the Medicaid expansion, they also experienced cross-pressures from the network of contributors and organizations associated with Charles Koch and recently deceased David Koch (Mayer 2017; Skocpol and Hertel-Fernandez 2016). These groups have enormous financial heft and have fought vigorously against state efforts to pass the Medicaid expansion (Skocpol and Hertel-Fernandez 2016). However, they are also active in fighting for conservative policy designs such as work requirements, and instituting copayment requirements on low-income Medicaid enrollees. This pressure was on full display in Kentucky when the newly elected Republican Governor Bevin wanted to overturn the Medicaid Expansion adopted under the previous Democratic governor. Because we conducted our interviews shortly after the election, respondents from Kentucky offered some important insights on the politics of the opioid epidemic in relation to the Medicaid program in their conservative state, which had moved to total Republican control. Several respondents described a fragmented Medicaid program under which the state could impose work requirements and, at the same time, embrace the program to address the opioid epidemic.

> He's pushing through a waiver that would allow him to do two things. One, he wants to charge at least like $10 a month as kind of a fee to Medicaid recipients and, two, he wants Medicaid recipients to show evidence of having gone back to work in order to retain their insurance . . . [since] we've got a Republican governor, a Republican Senate, and Republican House in this state right now; I don't really envision him having trouble getting that waiver through. He also wants to roll back the expansion but I don't think that's going to prove to be possible. (KY stakeholder no. 2, evaluation/research representative)

The majority of Republican voters in Kentucky and across the country support adopting the Medicaid expansion and, at the same time, conservative Medicaid policies such as copays and work requirements (Scott 2018). Some describe this as yet another paradox in US public opinion, but it is important to see the strategic Republican policy engineering reflected in holding these two views simultaneously.

The expand and retrench strategy among Republicans in Kentucky was described perfectly by stakeholders in the state. On the one level "Governor Bevin and his administration [will] need to provide treatment, [because] nobody is going to come out and say that they're against substance use treatment and everybody is moved by the stories of people dying." However, "at another level there's a lot of misgivings about government funding of services for [some] people" (KY stakeholder no. 8, Medicaid MCO representative). Republicans use Medicaid to address the opioid epidemic to appease their base, and use Medicaid to enact punitive policies targeted at groups deemed to be undeserving and most likely to vote for the Democratic party—"self-respecting people want the opportunity to work," said Governor Bevin.

By pursuing these conservative policy designs in their Medicaid programs, Kentucky and other Republican-led states used these conservative innovations (NH, IN, AR, and PA all pursued Medicaid waivers to adopt the

Medicaid expansion with conservative policy designs during the time period of our study [Grogan, Singer, and Jones, 2017]) to claim that their state was not adopting a *federal government*–run Medicaid program but their own private state version—despite drawing down more public funds than ever before. This is the strategic marketing that they hope will allow them to avoid blame from Tea Party groups who reject Medicaid.

Backstage Hidden Politics, Targeted Strategies: Medicaid Coverage Policy

Because states can leverage federal funds when they provide SUD treatment through Medicaid, utilizing the Medicaid program to finance SUD treatment is another important approach to address the opioid epidemic (NIDA 2016). It is also useful politically to Republican-led states that have openly rejected the Medicaid expansion, because coverage policy is largely hidden from public view.

The partisan politics of coverage policy is very different from the politics of the Medicaid expansion. While the Medicaid expansion is a highly salient political issue, coverage policy is characterized by pressure group politics where provider groups and advocates are very aware and pressure state legislators to expand benefits, but the general public is unaware (Grogan 1994; Miller et al. 2012). This hidden politics allows Republicans to expand coverage under Medicaid to target the needs of their base and of other key patient and provider stakeholders, without suffering any political repercussions from using a program they otherwise condemn.

Our 50-state survey of SUD benefits coverage reveals that although states with total Republican control are less likely to cover SUD benefits than other states with some Democratic representation, the percent of these states utilizing Medicaid to cover SUD benefits—especially individual, group, and intensive outpatient and detoxification services—is quite high in light of many officials' professed disdain for the program (see table 1).

It is important to point out the political context behind specific SUD treatments. First, methadone treatment has always been politically controversial. As a salient issue, it does not fit the usual "hidden politics" associated with coverage policy described above. This partisan divide is evident when we observe methadone coverage by state party control with only 64% of states with total Republican control covering methadone under Medicaid. While methadone coverage appears to reflect a partisan divide, the acceptance of other medications for OUD treatment among conservative states is remarkable and illustrates how states are using Medicaid coverage policy to implement targeted expansions for their own objectives and to appease stakeholders.

A Medicaid MCO representative from Georgia mentioned this shift in policy makers' thinking about addiction and those who suffer from it. "There's a framework shift happening in Georgia that . . . is moving us away from a punitive model related to substance use disorder, into a treatment focused . . . modality" (GA stakeholder no. 7). This framework shift in response to the opioid crisis is similar to that described above in Republican-led states that adopted the Medicaid expansion. What makes the ideological shift significant is that it happened at the same time that the state was openly rejecting the ACA Medicaid expansion. Indeed, according to our respondents, state policy makers were extremely resistant to anyone in state government even discussing the ACA or the Medicaid expansion. Georgia enacted the Georgia Health Care Freedom Act (HB 943), which forbids state government agencies from accepting or utilizing funding to advocate for any changes related to the ACA (*Georgia State University Law Review* 2014). Georgia stakeholders told us they were not allowed to mention the ACA or the Medicaid expansion in policy reports.

Given this, one might presume that Georgia would have been resistant to any Medicaid-related approaches to address the opioid epidemic. However, several respondents mentioned the broad range of SUD services that Medicaid covers in their state, and described continued efforts to expand services within Georgia's regular Medicaid program. A state agency representative mentioned that "if anything has Medicaid in front of it, we can't do it. That being said, very interestingly, we have extraordinary gubernatorial support on addiction, [and] he talks about people whose lives have really been turned around from *treatment*" (GA stakeholder no. 3). As a result, there is significant support for "addiction support services, drug [MAT] treatment, and community-based behavioral health services to be implemented [under Medicaid]" (GA stakeholder no. 3). What the stakeholders in Georgia described was a governor who eschews Medicaid when speaking to the public, but encourages state agencies to use Medicaid behind the scenes to cover medication treatment and other services to address the opioid epidemic. It is "that kind of the environment— mired in different and competing interests—" [that makes it] "very difficult to articulate" [what our] "priorities are" (GA stakeholder no. 3). And, that is the point of the strategy to keep it fragmented, diffuse, and confusing.

Although Florida did not adopt the ACA Medicaid expansion, the topic of Medicaid was not as politically sensitive as was described in Georgia.

Table 1 Percentage of States Requiring Medicaid Coverage of SUD Treatments and OUD Medications, 2017

Party control	N	Individual outpatient	Group outpatient	Intensive outpatient	Detox	Short-term residential
Total Republican	25	92%	96%	76%	80%	56%
Divided Republican governors	8	100%	100%	100%	100%	75%
Divided Democratic governors	11	100%	100%	82%	91%	73%
Total Democrats	6	100%	100%	100%	100%	83%
All states	50	96% (48)	98% (49)	84% (42)	88% (44)	66% (33)

Several respondents mentioned Senate Bill 12, which passed in April of 2016, as a major initiative to address behavioral health services generally, as well as the opioid epidemic. Florida's bill focused on improving the capacity of behavioral health providers by modifying licensure requirements making it possible to create a single, consolidated license to provide both mental health and substance use disorder services, and to create a coordinated system of care (Florida CS/SB 12—Mental Health and Substance Abuse Act, 2016).

While these aspects of the bill relied on state-only resources, it is significant that the legislation included a directive to the state Medicaid and Behavioral Health agencies to maximize federal Medicaid funding to cover services for behavioral health treatments. As a result, although several stakeholders mentioned SB12, respondents focused more on the importance of Medicaid maximization policies for addressing the opioid epidemic. "One of the things that we're mostly committed to . . . is really expanding access to Medicaid services for treatment" (FL stakeholder no. 1, state agency representative). A provider representative also described "this push to do revenue max. To use state money to draw down more Medicaid to serve more people in the mental health/substance abuse system" (FL stakeholder no. 5).

The targeted expand/retrench strategy also seems to have been written into SB12. As a state agency representative explained, state agencies are required to write a report to (1) identify the population it intends to target

Long-term residential	Recovery support services	Methadone	Oral Naltrexone	Injectable Naltrexone	Buprenorphine
36%	56%	64%	88%	92%	100%
50%	38%	100%	75%	75%	100%
55%	45%	82%	91%	91%	100%
83%	33%	100%	100%	100%	100%
48% (24)	48% (24)	78% (39)	88% (44)	90% (45)	100% (50)

and whether the state should (or can) expand eligibility in any way, (2) define coverage policy for the target, and (3) specify a process and a plan for how the state would be able to meet the needs specified through revenue maximization (FL stakeholder no. 6). And, they definitely view persons with OUD—and providers who serve this population—as a target for expansion. "We are looking at our appropriations to reallocate some of our funding to make sure that we direct more funding to the treatment of those [with OUD] who need medication treatment" (FL stakeholder no. 7, state agency representative).

Another important pattern among state party control and Medicaid SUD coverage policy emerges with residential treatment. Under Section 1905(a)(B) of the Social Security Act (the Institution for Mental Diseases exclusion), the federal government did not allow financial support for Medicaid coverage of SUD residential treatment. However, just in the last couple years, states can apply for a waiver to cover residential services in large part to address demand for such services among SUD providers and some people living with OUD. This is a major commitment from the federal government and any state that takes up the benefit, because residential treatment is very expensive. Given the Republican Party's commitment to lowering taxes, it is perhaps not surprising that states under total Republic control have been less eager than states under Democrat control to offer the benefit (see table 1).

Nonetheless, it is noteworthy that more than half (14) of the states with total Republican control cover this expensive benefit in their Medicaid programs to target the opioid crisis. Florida, for example, submitted a Medicaid waiver to the federal government specifically to expand Medicaid covered SUD residential treatment services, and also focused on building SUD provider participation in the Medicaid program.

State coverage of recovery support services also reveals an important pattern. Recovery support is a relatively new Medicaid covered service enacted in response to the opioid epidemic. The federal government allows states to cover the service with a federal financial match. This is the one SUD benefit in which states under total Republican control are *more* likely than Democrat-controlled states to provide coverage under Medicaid (see table 1).

Several reasons may help to account for this. First, recovery support services include a range of nonclinical services that may address the individual's environment, such as supportive housing or employment, and/ or provide emotional and practical support to maintain remission. The latter services typically include peer support, such as individual mentoring or peer-led support groups. Although the federal government will pay for the range of recovery support services, most states only pay for peer supports (McMullen 2019). While housing and employment supports are costly, payments for peer support are relatively modest.

Second, peer-led recovery support services can also be conceptualized as a service that promotes individual behavioral modification and personal responsibility and can be structured as a faith-based program, which fits well with a conservative ideology and has been heavily emphasized in conservative policy designs adopted by Republican-led states (Grogan, Singer, and Jones 2017). This kind of individual-based ideology can be seen in Georgia's Recovery Transformation Program, a major initiative that utilizes persons who have experience with addiction as peer workers (or peer coaches) to help people with OUD.

> Recovery transformation means that the State Department of Behavioral Health [has] really embraced a concept that recovery starts from a position of a client themselves; . . . recovery services . . . up until recently, was top down. A client would come into our system and . . . be handed over to a therapist, who then gave instruction to a client. Now, we're trying to . . . deliver person-centered recovery services with a big emphasis on peers. That has really happened over the last two to three years. (GA Stakeholder NO. 4, provider representative)

The Recovery Transformation Project is also viewed as a method for developing workforce capacity in Georgia. "This is a workforce development initiative for us," [the director of the state agency] "wanted a peer workforce" (GA stakeholder no. 2, recovery policy advocate). It is important to see how conservative ideology fits with this preference for peer-delivered recovery support services: it encourages an individual responsibility frame, and relying on a peer workforce is relatively inexpensive and can also be used to delegitimize formal SUD services, especially those that rely heavily on government funding. Within the context of Medicaid expansion and other health care policy reforms, peer-delivered recovery support services are also covered in liberal states, but are often considered as part of a comprehensive continuum of care, complementary to formal SUD treatment (Bersamira 2018). In contrast, when Republican-led states conceptualize peer support as individual responsibility, it can be considered as in alignment with other conservative policy designs, such as incentives for healthy lifestyles.

Symbolic Politics: State Opioid-Related Legislation

We turn now to analyze what type of opioid-related legislation states have proposed and enacted, and whether there are differences by state party control. Between 2014 and 2018, 1,804 pieces of legislation related to opioids were introduced across all 50 states. Given the severity of the opioid epidemic, legislatures in all states—regardless of party control—proposed legislation to address this issue. Of those introduced, 497 were eventually enacted.

Policy Approaches to Address Opioids

Opioid-related legislation was divided into ten different categories (see table 2). Across all opioid-related policy types, more than half of the states introduced legislation. Every state introduced legislation that would raise awareness about opioid use and the opioid epidemic. "Raising Awareness" was also the most frequent approach to be enacted in state legislatures with 43 states enacting this type of legislation. Because the fiscal impact of this type of legislation is relatively less costly ($131,000 on average) compared to the other legislative options proposed and enacted, this emphasis by state policy makers is not surprising (see table 3). Although some states mandated school curricula to address opioid use and misuse in secondary

Table 2 Legislative Policies Addressing Opioid Epidemic by States, Votes, and Party, 2014–18

Policy examples	Regulating prescription drug monitoring programs	Regulating pain management clinics	Increasing naloxone access	Regulating legal system and opioids
No. of states with legislation introduced	50	30	46	36
No. of states with legislation enacted	41	17	41	22
Floor votes for nonenacted legislation	93%	93%	95%	97%
Republicans	90%	90%	92%	98%
Democrats	97%	99%	99%	96%
Floor votes for enacted legislation	97%	99%	98%	96%
Republicans	97%	99%	98%	95%
Democrats	98%	99%	99%	97%

and/or higher education, it was common to raise awareness through less intensive efforts, either by declaring a pain awareness or prescription pill awareness day or week within the state, which are obviously relatively inexpensive options.

All states introduced and the majority (41) enacted more intensive legislation to establish prescription drug monitoring programs (PDMPs), which mandate the collection and analysis of opioid prescription utilization data. This is noteworthy because the PDMP approach is organizationally complex and costly ($330,000 on average) relative to the other approaches enacted. Legislation that would increase access to naloxone for either the general public or first responders was also common, with 46 states introducing and 41 enacting such legislation. These measures also often involved more substantial fiscal commitment and government action relative to other options.

Partisan Voting Patterns within States

An analysis of the voting patterns on proposed and enacted legislation addressing opioids highlights largely bipartisan support at the state level. Overall, 96% of votes by Democrats and Republicans across all the states

Regulating immunity laws	Regulating prescriptions	Regulating workforce	Raising awareness	Non-MAT prevention approaches	Regulating insurance products
39	43	45	50	38	34
33	31	32	43	29	17
93%	95%	93%	95%	89%	99%
90%	92%	92%	94%	84%	99%
96%	99%	93%	96%	95%	99%
99%	97%	98%	97%	95%	93%
98%	98%	97%	98%	91%	94%
99%	97%	99%	97%	99%	92%

were in support of some type of opioid legislation. The level of support by the type of legislation is also very similar for enacted legislation (see table 2). For legislation that was not enacted, only nonmedication prevention approaches dipped below 90% of support by Republicans, who were more likely to oppose compared to their Democratic counterparts. Nonmedication prevention approaches focus on politically controversial opioid prevention strategies like needle exchanges, safe injection sites, and (less controversially) drug take-back programs.

Although we observe bipartisan support for proposed and enacted legislation, it is important to note that the policies that make it onto the political agenda are subject to the "mobilization of bias" that E. E. Schattschneider ([1960] 1975) famously describes. Although we did not collect data on the agenda-setting process, it is almost certainly the case that particular policy proposals were denied access to the legislative agenda because they were perceived as too costly, such as any policy providing OUD treatment, or too partisan, such as any proposal related to the ACA, making passage unlikely (see also Bachrach and Baratz 1962). As Richard L. Hall and Frank W. Wayman's (1990) foundational study of the role of money in politics illustrates, focusing on floor votes occludes a great deal of politics that occurs behind the scenes. They find that committee bargaining is the

Table 3 Fiscal Analysis of Opioid Legislation by Policy Domain

Policy examples	Regulating prescription drug monitoring programs	Regulating pain management clinics	Increasing naloxone access	Regulating legal system and opioids
Average fiscal impact on introduced legislation (enacted legislation	$607,242 ($330,590)	$800,198 ($2,089,669)	$105,159 ($208,896)	$748,790 ($288,992)
Per capita fiscal impact of introduced legislation (enacted legislation)	$0.17 ($0.32)	$0.04 ($0.26)	$0.01 ($0.02)	$0.51 ($0.14)
Percentage of total state appropriations of introduced legislation (enacted legislation)	0.01% (0.01%)	0.002% (0.01%)	0.0002% (0.0008%)	0.02% (0.008%)

real driver in terms of influencing what ends up in legislation, and all this happens prior to bills arriving on the floor for a vote.

Some states with total Republican Party control have openly rejected the Medicaid expansion and yet face significant public pressure to address the opioid epidemic. Do these states pass legislation that is different in content or fiscal commitment from Democrat-led states that have passed the Medicaid expansion? Although Republican-led states have actively passed non-Medicaid legislation to address the opioid epidemic, none of the ten major pieces of the legislation offered access to OUD treatment, as is provided through Medicaid expansion. In the domain of harm reduction, naloxone is not only an important life-saving emergency treatment but also a stop-gap measure especially when viewed against the recommended OUD treatment package the helps a person move toward recovery.

Fiscal Analysis of Opioid Policies

Not surprisingly, the average fiscal impact across the states for different policy approaches varied quite substantially: ranging from a low of about $11,000 for regulating prescriptions, which primarily entails data reporting

Regulating immunity laws	Regulating prescriptions	Regulating workforce	Raising awareness	Non-MAT prevention approaches	Regulating insurance products
$28,767	$577,307	$32,817	$301,620	$889,330	$763,911
($56,146)	($10,869)	($72,408)	($131,121)	($234,719)	($15,506)
<$0.00	$0.10	<$0.00	$0.04	$0.21	$0.10
($0.01)	(<$0.01)	($0.02)	($0.03)	($0.04)	($0.01)
<0.0001%	0.004%	<0.0001%	0.001%	0.005%	0.003%
(<0.0001%)	(<0.0001%)	(<0.0001%)	(0.001%)	(0.001%)	(<0.0001%)

requirements, to a high of $2,000,000 for regulating pain management clinics (see table 3). To control for the fact that appropriations will naturally be higher in larger, more prosperous states (i.e., New York and California), we calculated the per capita fiscal impact and the percent of the fiscal impact based on total state appropriations. These measures reveal that regulating PDMPs is not only one of the most frequently enacted legislative approaches to address the opioid epidemic but also the second most costly (see table 3).

State Party Control by Legislative Type and Fiscal Impact

States with total party control were more likely to enact opioid-related legislation than states with divided partisan control (see table 4). However, there is little difference between total Republican- and total Democrat-controlled states in the most frequent legislative approaches—PDMP, increasing naloxone access, and raising awareness are similarly the three most popular approaches across party control. It is noteworthy, given Republican's distrustful rhetoric regarding government regulation, that it is much more common in Republican-controlled states to enact regulating

Table 4 Average Fiscal Impact of Enacted Opioid Legislation by Policy Domain and Political Party

Party control	N	Regulating prescription drug monitoring programs	Regulating pain management clinics	Increasing naloxone access	Regulating legal system and opioids
Total	31	26 (22)	16 (10)	25 (22)	18 (12)
Republican		71%	32%	71%	39%
Divided	7	5 (3)	2 (1)	5 (5)	3 (1)
Republican governors		43%	14%	71%	14%
Divided	9	6 (4)	4 (1)	6 (4)	7 (4)
Democratic governors		45%	11%	44%	44%
Total	14	13 (12)	8 (5)	10 (10)	8 (5)
Democrat		86%	36%	71%	36%

immunity laws than it is in Democratic-controlled states (71% compared to 36%).[2] However, Democrat-controlled states are more likely to enact legislation that provides nonmedication prevention and that regulates insurance products.

The average fiscal impact of opioid-related legislation in Republican-controlled states is substantially less than in Democratic-controlled states (see table 5a). Overall, Republican-controlled states spent about $95,000 on average for opioid-related legislation compared to about $278,000 in Democratic-controlled states.

States are constrained by many factors and histories independent of opioid-specific concerns. States' fiscal policies are shaped by path dependencies such that the amount of revenue available to them is the result of past taxation policies, the strength of the state's economy, and spending on other issues. Consequently, the decisions that set a state down a certain fiscal policy path may have been made under a government whose partisan makeup differed from the present configuration. Nonetheless, the vast majority of the total Republican-controlled states have been controlled by the Republican Party for a long time: 9 states have been under total Republican control for the last 10 years, and an additional 12 have at least

2. However, see Miller et al. 2012 for similar partisan finding regarding Medicaid Wage Pass-through Adoption.

Regulating immunity laws	Regulating prescriptions	Regulating workforce	Raising awareness	Non-MAT prevention approaches	Regulating insurance products
24 (22)	23 (17)	24 (18)	27 (24)	19 (15)	17 (8)
71%	55%	58%	75%	48%	26%
4 (3)	4 (2)	5 (4)	4 (3)	3 (2)	2 (2)
43%	29%	57%	43%	29%	29%
4 (3)	5 (3)	5 (2)	5 (4)	5 (4)	4 (1)
33%	33%	22%	44%	44%	11%
7 (5)	11 (9)	11 (8)	14 (12)	11 (8)	11 (6)
36%	64%	57%	88%	57%	43%

been under Republican legislative (Senate and House) control while having a Republican governor for the entire 10-year period. Thus, these states might have been constrained by past Republican Party decisions in their state, but not by the Democratic Party. Yet, it is certainly the case that states are constrained by the strength of their economy; obviously, it is difficult to have a high-tax effort when the revenue base is low. Moreover, less-populous states may spend less because they have different needs or more limited OUD treatment infrastructures. For these reasons, we calculate per capita fiscal impact to adjust for population size across the states, and percent of total appropriations spent to compare what states spend on opioid legislation relative to the total base of their commitments.

When we focus on these measures, we find the same average per capita fiscal commitment for all opioid legislation across states with different party control (see first column in table 5b). However, when we look at percent of total appropriations, states under total Republican control devote a higher proportion of their state spending to opioid-related legislation than states under total Democrat control (see table 5c).

As we look across both measures, Republican-controlled states spend more per capita and devote more of their resources on the following six legislative approaches: regulating pain management clinics, regulating legal

Table 5a Average Fiscal Impact of Enacted Opioid Legislation by Policy Domain and Political Party

Party control	N	All opioid policies	Regulating prescription drug monitoring programs	Regulating pain management clinics	Increasing naloxone access	Regulating legal system and opioids
Total	31	$421,166	$424,821	$141,314	$31,464	$221,428
Republican		($95,352)	($19,522)	($281,107)	($25,572)	($139,600)
Divided	7	$964,739	$0	$2,200,000	$0	$9,994,500
Republican governors		($67,446)	($120,000)	($0)	($10,428)	($0)
Divided	9	$302,653	$6,237	$0	$13,043	$997,333
Democratic governors		($174,000)	($18,666)	($0)	($50,000)	($1,905,000)
Total	14	$1,376,243	$251,059	$0	$110,032	$0
Democrat		($278,303)	($37,284)	($0)	($63,000)	($0)

Table 5b Per-Capita Fiscal Impact of Enacted Opioid Legislation by Policy Domain and Political Party

Party control	N	All opioid policies	Regulating prescription drug monitoring programs	Regulating pain management clinics	Increasing naloxone access	Regulating legal system and opioids
Total		$0.06	$0.07	$0.02	$0.01	$0.03
Republican		($0.02)	(<$0.00)	($0.07)	($0.01)	($0.02)
Divided		$0.07	$0	$1.05	$0	$7.47
Republican governors		($0.02)	($0.06)	($0)	(<$0.01)	($0)
Divided		$0.03	<$0.01	$0	<$0.01	$0.23
Democrat governors		($0.09)	(<$0.01)	($0)	(<$0.01)	($1.03)
Total		$0.19	$0.03	$0	$0.01	$0
Democrat		($0.02)	($0.01)	($0)	(<$0.01)	($0)

Regulating immunity laws	Regulating prescriptions	Regulating workforce	Raising awareness	Non-MAT prevention approaches	Regulating insurance products
$4,666	$1,119,776	$860	$565,502	$61,405	$3,315
($82,567)	($26,887)	($34,200)	($117,950)	($510,757)	($266)
$0	$0	$0	$0	$0	$0
($0)	($0)	($403,180)	($0)	($0)	($0)
$0	$0	$0	$712,962	$0	$0
($0)	($0)	($5,000)	($0)	($0)	($0)
$0	$1,461,692	$86,306	$400,904	$3,142,865	$0
($0)	($0)	($49,732)	($244,189)	($133,926)	($0)

Regulating immunity laws	Regulating prescriptions	Regulating workforce	Raising awareness	Non-MAT prevention approaches	Regulating insurance products
<$0.01	$0.19	<$0.01	$0.06	$0.01	<$0.01
($0.01)	($0.01)	($0.01)	($0.06)	($0.08)	(<$0.01)
$0	$0	$0	$0	$0	$0
($0)	($0)	($0.09)	($0)	($0)	($0)
$0	$0	$0	$0.04	$0	$0
($0)	($0)	(<$0.01)	($0)	($0)	($0)
$0	$0.20	$0.01	$0.07	$0.06	$0
($0)	($0)	($0.01)	($0.04)	($0.02)	($0)

Table 5c Percent of Total State Appropriations of Enacted Opioid Legislation by Policy Domain and Political Party

Party control	N	All opioid policies	Regulating prescription drug monitoring programs	Regulating pain management clinics	Increasing naloxone access	Regulating legal system and opioids
Total		0.003%	0.005%	<0.0001%	<0.0001%	0.001%
Republican		(0.001%)	(<0.0001%)	(0.004%)	(<0.0001%)	(<0.0001%)
Divided		0.03%	0%	0.04%	0%	0.28%
Republican governor		(<0.0001%)	(0.002%)	(0%)	(0.002%)	(0%)
Divided		0.001%	<0.0001%	0%	<0.0001%	0.01%
Democrat governors		(0.004%)	(0.0001%)	(0%)	(<0.0001%)	(0.04%)
Total		0.006%	0.001%	0%	<0.0001%	0%
Democrat		(0.0006%)	(<0.0001%)	(0%)	(<0.0001%)	(0%)

system and opioids, regulating immunity laws, regulating prescriptions, nonmedication prevention approaches, and regulating insurance products (see tables 5b and 5c).

In sum, it is noteworthy that Republican-controlled states are active in using state government to address the opioid epidemic—over 50% of these states enacted 6 of the 10 legislative approaches, and devoted a higher proportion of their own public resources to these opioid-related initiatives.

It is equally important to note what these states did *not* do: none of the 10 legislative approaches provide access to OUD *treatment*. The lack of extending government support for access to OUD treatment has consequences. Uninsured adults with OUD are much less likely than someone with private insurance or Medicaid coverage to receive treatment (Wu, Zhu, and Swartz 2016). Low-income uninsured adults in states that have not expanded Medicaid—all Republican-controlled states—are less likely to gain coverage and access to affordable treatment for OUD (Clemans-Cope et al. 2019). In contrast, coverage of medications for OUD, considered necessary for recovery, has been growing in expansion states (Miller 2018; SAMHSA 2018).

For states that adopt the Medicaid expansion and provide OUD medications, the financial commitment is enormous. Because the number of

Regulating immunity laws	Regulating prescriptions	Regulating workforce	Raising awareness	Non-MAT prevention approaches	Regulating insurance products
<0.0001%	0.01%	<0.0001%	0.004%	0.0004%	<0.0001%
(0.001%)	(<0.0001%)	(<0.0001%)	(0.003%)	(0.004%)	(<0.0001%)
0%	0%	0%	0% (0%)	0%	0%
(0%)	(0%)	(0.004%)		(0%)	(0%)
0%	0%	0%	0.001%	0%	0%
(0%)	(0%)	(<0.0001%)	(0%)	(0%)	(0%)
0%	0.007%	0.0003%	0.002%	0.02%	0%
(0%)	(0%)	(0.0002%)	(0.002)	(0.0007%)	(0%)

prescriptions for OUD in expansion states far exceeds nonexpansion states (e.g., 170 prescriptions per 1,000 Medicaid enrollees for buprenorphine in late-expansion states compared to 30 in nonexpansion states), the difference in spending is substantial. For buprenorphine alone, expansion states spent $607 million in 2017 compared to $80 million in nonexpansion states (Cope). Comparing spending on state opioid-related legislative actions to that spent on just one OUD medication (this does not include all the other treatments listed in table 1) illustrates the symbolic politics behind the Republican-led state-level legislative approach.

Conclusion: Republican Policies for Addressing the Opioid Epidemic—Active but Meager

Republican opposition to the Medicaid expansion and the ACA has been deep and persistent. Moreover, the unwillingness of most states under total Republican control to pull the biggest lever—adopting the Medicaid expansion—means that even when these states attempt to maximize federal revenue in their regular Medicaid programs to address the opioid epidemic, the amount of federal funding they can ultimately draw down for OUD treatment was (and continues to be) quite modest in comparison to those states that have expanded.

In 2017, nearly 20 million people with OUD needed treatment. The vast majority did not receive it, many because they couldn't afford it (Gebelhoff 2018). Given that many of those directly affected by the opioid epidemic live in areas of dominant Republican Party control and sometimes reflect core Republican constituencies, why aren't those who are not obtaining treatment holding the party responsible?

Time will tell, but it appears for now that the Republican strategy of embracing a conservative welfare state, which includes targeted expansion and retrenchment at the state-level, has been an effective strategy to avoid blame and serve key stakeholders.

Many of these state-level initiatives are valuable reforms. Republican officeholders will surely cite them in their campaigns to demonstrate that the GOP is still capable of working across the aisle and passing major legislation. Yet, the details behind state-level initiatives puncture illusions of bipartisanship in a public health emergency. Medications and outpatient services are necessary, evidence-based treatment services to address OUD (NIDA 2016). Although Republican nonexpansion strategies might work politically, these fail to address a raging epidemic, leaving many Americans without access to life-saving treatment.

■ ■ ■

Colleen M. Grogan is a professor at the University of Chicago in the School of Social Service Administration. Her research interests include health policy, health politics, and the American welfare state. She has written extensively on the history and current politics of the US Medicaid program. She also is completing a book manuscript titled *The Rise of America's Conservative Health Care State*, which examines the historical development of political strategies and motivations behind hiding the expanding role of government in the US health care system. She is associate editor for the health policy section of the *American Journal of Public Health*. cgrogan@uchicago.edu

Clifford S. Bersamira is an assistant professor at the University of Hawai'i at Mānoa Myron B. Thompson School of Social Work. He is the principal investigator for Hawai'i CARES, the state's program funded by the Department of Health, Alcohol and Drug Abuse Division, to develop a statewide single-entry care coordination system for substance use disorder treatment. He received his PhD and AM (MSW equivalent) from the University of Chicago and a BA from the University of Pennsylvania. Previously he provided technical assistance to state governments and conducted policy research with the National Association of State Alcohol and Drug Abuse Directors.

Phillip M. Singer is an assistant professor in the Department of Political Science at the University of Utah. His research focuses on state health policy and politics, comparative social policy, and implementation of the Affordable Care Act.

Bikki Tran Smith is currently a fifth-year doctoral candidate in social work at the University of Chicago. Her broad research interest explores the intersection of race, place, health, and health policy. She has conducted more than 10 years of research and practice combined in the areas of behavioral health, health policy, housing, homelessness, disabilities, and technology in the classroom.

Harold A. Pollack is the Helen Ross Professor of Social Service Administration and an affiliate professor in the Biological Sciences Collegiate Division and Department of Public Health Sciences at the University of Chicago. He is codirector of the University of Chicago Health Lab and the University of Chicago Crime Lab. His current research concerns interventions to serve individuals living with substance use or psychiatric disorders who come into contact with law enforcement and correctional systems.

Christina M. Andrews is an associate professor at the College of Social Work at the University of South Carolina. Her research focuses on strategies to increase access to opioid-use disorder treatment. She has conducted extensive research on the role of the Affordable Care Act in improving access to addiction treatment. She is principal investigator of a five-year Research Scientist Development Award from the National Institute on Drug Abuse to assess the effectiveness of Medicaid health homes in treating addiction and reducing the need for acute care for addiction-related conditions. She received her doctoral degree from the University of Chicago.

Amanda J. Abraham is an associate professor of public administration and policy in the School of Public and International Affairs at the University of Georgia. Her research focuses on the impact of federal and state policy on the accessibility and quality of substance use disorder treatment and the adoption, diffusion, and implementation of evidence-based practices for the treatment of substance use disorder, organizational change, and workforce development. She currently serves as principal investigator and coinvestigator on numerous federal grants funded by the National Institute on Drug Abuse, the Substance Abuse and Mental Health Services Administration, and the US Department of Agriculture.

Acknowledgments

This research was supported by the Center for Health Administration Studies at the University of Chicago. We acknowledge research assistance from Geoff Clark and very helpful comments from workshop participants at Brown University and from an anonymous reviewer for *JHPPL*. We also gratefully acknowledge the participation of state stakeholders in the state case study portion of this research.

References

Altarum. 2018. "Economic Toll of Opioid Crisis in the US Exceeded $1 Trillion since 2001." Newsroom, February 13. altarum.org/news/economic-toll-opioid-crisis-us -exceeded-1-trillion-2001.

Bachrach, Peter, and Morton S. Baratz. 1962. "Two Faces of Power." *American Political Science Review* 56, no. 4: 947–52.

Barrilleaux, Charles, and Carlisle Rainey. 2014. "The Politics of Need: Examining Governors' Decisions to Oppose the 'Obamacare' Medicaid Expansion." *State Politics and Policy Quarterly* 14, no. 4: 437–60.

Bersamira, Clifford S. 2018. "Policy Stakeholder Perspectives on Addiction Recovery in the Era of Healthcare Reform." PhD diss., University of Chicago.

Bonica, Adam. 2013. "Ideology and Interests in the Political Marketplace." *American Journal of Political Science* 57, no. 2: 294–311.

Clemans-Cope, Lisa, Marni Epstein, Victoria Lynch, and Emma Winiski. 2019. "Rapid Growth in Medicaid Spending and Prescriptions to Treat Opioid Use Disorder and Opioid Overdose from 2010 to 2017." Urban Institute Health Policy Center, February. urban.org/sites/default/files/publication/99798/rapid_growth_in _medical_spending_and_prescriptions_to_treat_opioid_use_disorder_and_opioid _overdose_from_2010_to_2017_1.pdf.

Florida State Senate. 2016. *Mental Health and Substance Abuse Act.* SB 12. 114th Cong., 2nd sess. Introduced January 7. www.flsenate.gov/Session/Bill/2016/0012 (accessed October 23, 2019).

Gebelhoff, Robert. 2018. "Don't Be Fooled. Republicans Don't Care about the Opioid Epidemic." *Washington Post*, September 17. www.washingtonpost.com/blogs/post -partisan/wp/2018/09/17/dont-be-fooled-republicans-dont-care-about-the-opioid -epidemic/.

Georgia State University Law Review. 2014. "Georgia Health Care Freedom Act HB 943." *Georgia State University Law Review* 31, no. 1: 112–28. readingroom.law .gsu.edu/gsulr/vol31/iss1/7 (accessed October 23, 2019).

Goodwin, James S., Yong-Fang Kuo, David Brown, David Juurlink, and Mukaila Raji. 2018. "Association of Chronic Opioid Use with Presidential Voting Patterns in US Counties in 2016." *JAMA Network Open* 1, no. 2: e180450. doi.org/10.1001/ jamanetworkopen.2018.0450.

Grogan, Colleen M. 1994. "The Political-Economic Factors Influencing State Medicaid Policy." *Political Research Quarterly* 47, no. 3: 589–622.

Grogan, Colleen M. 2014. "Medicaid: Designed to Grow." In *Health Politics and Policy*, 5th ed., edited by James A. Morone and Daniel C. Ehlke, 142–63. Stamford, CT: Cengage Learning.

Grogan, Colleen M., Christina Andrews, Amanda Abraham, Keith Humphreys, Harold A. Pollack, Bikki Tran Smith, and Peter D. Friedmann. 2016. "Survey Highlights Differences in Medicaid Coverage for Substance Use Treatment and Opioid Use Disorder Medications." *Health Affairs* 35, no. 12: 2289–96.

Grogan, Colleen M., and Eric M. Patashnik. 2003. "Between Welfare Medicine and Mainstream Entitlement: Medicaid at the Political Crossroads." *Journal of Health Politics, Policy and Law* 28 no. 5: 821–58.

Grogan, Colleen M., and Peter D. Jacobson, eds. 2013. "The Supreme Court's PPACA Decision." Special Section, *Journal of Health Politics, Policy and Law* 38, no. 2: 225–98.

Grogan, Colleen M., Phillip M. Singer, and David K. Jones. 2017. "Rhetoric and Reform in Waiver States." *Journal of Health Politics, Policy and Law* 42, no. 2: 247–84.

Grogan, Colleen M., and Sunggeun Park. 2017. "The Racial Divide in State Medicaid Expansions." *Journal of Health Politics, Policy and Law* 42, no. 3: 539–72.

Grogan, Colleen M., and Sunggeun Park. 2018. "Medicaid Retrenchment Politics: Fragmented or Unified?" *Journal of Social Policy and Aging* 30, nos. 3–4: 372–99.

Hacker, Jacob S., and Paul Pierson. 2015. "Confronting Asymmetric Polarization." In *Solutions to Political Polarization in America*, edited by Nathaniel Persily, 59–70. Cambridge: Cambridge University Press.

Hacker, Jacob S., and Paul Pierson. 2018. "The Dog That Almost Barked: What the ACA Repeal Fight Says about the Resilience of the American Welfare State." *Journal of Health Politics, Policy and Law* 43, no. 4: 551–77.

Hall, Richard L., and Frank W. Wayman. 1990. "Buying Time: Moneyed Interests and the Mobilization of Bias in Congressional Committees." *American Political Science Review* 84, no. 3: 797–820.

Johnson, Travis. 2017. "Americans Think Opioid Addiction Is a Crisis. They're Not Sure Federal Dollars Will Solve It." *Washington Post*, August 10. www .washingtonpost.com/news/monkey-cage/wp/2017/08/09/americans-think-opioid -addiction-is-a-crisis-theyre-not-sure-federal-dollars-will-solve-it/.

KFF (Henry J. Kaiser Family Foundation). n.d. "Medicaid Expansion Enrollment." State Health Facts. kff.org/health-reform/state-indicator/medicaid-expansion -enrollment/ (accessed January 14, 2020).

Kliff, Sarah. 2016. "Why Obamacare Enrollees Voted for Trump." *Vox*, December 13. www.vox.com/science-and-health/2016/12/13/13848794/kentucky-obamacare -trump.

Kliff, Sarah. 2017. "The Opioid Crisis Changed How Doctors Think about Pain." *Vox*, June 5. www.vox.com/2017/6/5/15111936/opioid-crisis-pain-west-virginia.

Lanford, Daniel, and Jill Quadagno. 2016. "Implementing Obamacare: The Politics of Medicaid Expansion under the Affordable Care Act of 2010." *Sociological Perspectives* 59, no. 3: 619–39.

Mann, Thomas E., and Norman J. Ornstein. 2013. "Finding the Common Good in an Era of Dysfunctional Governance." *Daedalus* 142, no. 2: 15–24.

Mayer, Jane. 2017. *Dark Money: The Hidden History of the Billionaires behind the Rise of the Radical Right*. New York: Anchor Books.

McMullen, Erin K. 2019. "Recovery Support Services for Medicaid Beneficiaries with a Substance Use Disorder." Medicaid and CHIP Payment and Access Commission, March. macpac.gov/publication/recovery-support-services-for-medicaid -beneficiaries-with-substance-use-disorder/.

Miller, Edward Alan, Lili Wang, Zhanlian Feng, and Vincent Mor. 2012. "Improving Direct-Care Compensation in Nursing Homes: Medicaid Wage Pass-Through Adoption, 1999–2004." *Journal of Health Politics, Policy and Law* 37, no. 3: 469–512.

NIDA (National Institute on Drug Abuse). 2016. "Effective Treatments for Opioid Addiction." November. www.drugabuse.gov/publications/effective-treatments-opioid -addiction/effective-treatments-opioid-addiction.

O'Donnell, Julie K., R. Matthew Gladden, and Puja Seth. 2017. "Trends in Deaths Involving Heroin and Synthetic Opioids Excluding Methadone, and Law Enforcement Drug Product Reports, by Census Region—United States, 2006–2015." *Morbidity and Mortality Weekly Report* 66, no. 34: 897–903.

Patashnik, Eric M., and Jonathan Oberlander. 2018. "After Defeat: Conservative Postenactment Opposition to the ACA in Historical-Institutional Perspective." *Journal of Health Politics, Policy and Law* 43, no. 4: 651–82.

Politico/Harvard T. H. Chan School of Public Health Poll. 2018. "Americans' Views on Policies to Address Prescription Drug Prices, the Opioid Crisis, and Other Current Domestic Issues." July 2. static.politico.com/50/19/6924fa8d4f238f1b9fc 155a275a3/drug-pricing-poll.pdf.

Rosenbaum, Sara. 2012. "Threading the Needle—Medicaid and the 113th Congress." *New England Journal of Medicine* 367, no. 25: 2368–69.

Rudd, Rose A., Puja Seth, Felicita David, and Lawrence Scholl. 2016. "Increases in Drug and Opioid-Involved Overdose Deaths—United States, 2010–2015." *Morbidity and Mortality Weekly Report* 65, nos. 50–51: 1445–52.

Sabatier, Paul A., and Christopher M. Weible. 2007. "The Advocacy Coalition: Innovations and Clarifications." In *Theories of the Policy Process*, 2nd ed., edited by Paul A. Sabatier, 189–220. Boulder, CO: Westview Press.

SAMHSA (Substance Abuse and Mental Health Services Administration). 2018. "Medicaid Coverage of Medication-Assisted Treatment for Alcohol and Opioid Use Disorders and of Medication for the Reversal of Opioid Overdose." SMA18-5093, November. store.samhsa.gov/product/Medicaid-Coverage-of-Medication -Assisted-Treatment-for-Alcohol-and-Opioid-Use-Disorders-and-of-Medication -for-the-Reversal-of-Opioid-Overdose/SMA18-5093.

Schattschneider, Elmer E., and David Adamany. (1960) 1975. *The Semisovereign People: A Realist's View of Democracy in America*. Rev. ed. Boston: Cengage Learning.

Scholl, Lawrence, Puja Seth, Mbabazi Kariisa, Nana Otoo Wilson, and Grant Baldwin. 2018. "Drug and Opioid-Involved Overdose Deaths—United States, 2013–2017." *Morbidity and Mortality Weekly Report* 67, no. 5152: 1419–27.

Scott, Dylan. 2018. "America's Medicaid Work Requirement Paradox, Explained by Two Polls." *Vox*, February 5. www.vox.com/health-care/2018/2/5/16975574 /medicaid-work-requirement-paradox-polls.

Segel, Joel E., Yunfeng Shi, John R. Moran, and Dennis P. Scanlon. 2019. "Revenue Losses to State and Federal Government from Opioid-Related Employment Reductions." *Medical Care* 57, no. 7: 494–97.

Skocpol, Theda, and Alexander Hertel-Fernandez. 2016. "The Koch Network and Republican Party Extremism." *Perspectives on Politics* 14, no. 3: 681–99.

Skocpol, Theda, and Lawrence R. Jacobs, eds. 2011. *Reaching for a New Deal: Ambitious Governance, Economic Meltdown, and Polarized Politics in Obama's First Two Years.* New York: Russell Sage Foundation.

Smith, Mitch. 2018. "What Do These Political Ads Have in Common? The Opioid Crisis." *New York Times*, June 7. www.nytimes.com/2018/06/07/us/opioid-ads -democrats-republicans.html.

Weiss, Robert S. 1995. *Learning From Strangers: The Art and Method of Qualitative Interview Studies.* New York: Free Press.

Wu, Li-Tzy, He Zhu, and Marvin S. Swartz. 2016. "Treatment Utilization among Persons with Opioid Use Disorder in the United States." *Drug and Alcohol Dependence* 169: 117–27.

Public Preferences for New Information on Opioids

Paul F. Testa
Susan L. Moffitt
Marie Schenk
Brown University

Abstract

Context: Educating the public through information campaigns is a commonly used policy approach to public health problems. Yet, experimental methods that assess the impact of information campaigns may misestimate their effects by failing to account for respondents' willingness to receive new information.

Methods: This article uses a doubly randomized survey experiment conducted on a nationally representative sample, where some subjects are randomly assigned to an informational treatment about opioids while other subjects are given the choice of whether to receive treatment or not, to examine how public willingness to seek new information shapes the way they update their preferences about policies related to the opioid epidemic.

Findings: Among those likely to receive information, treatment has a large positive effect on increasing support for policies that address the opioid epidemic by about one half of a standard deviation. Among those who would avoid this information, preferences appear to be unmoved by treatment. These effects would be missed by standard experimental designs.

Conclusion: While redressing information asymmetries is only one part of a public health strategy for addressing the opioid epidemic, our findings highlight the importance of access to and receptiveness toward new information.

Keywords   opioid epidemic, public health, information campaigns

Knowledge problems pervade the US opioid epidemic. Health professionals face continued uncertainty in understanding, assessing, and treating patient pain, especially chronic noncancer pain (Bonnie et al. 2019; IOM 2011; NAS 2017).[1] Regulators and health professionals face ongoing

---

1. On physician payments and associations with opioid prescriptions, see Hadland et al. 2019.

Journal of Health Politics, Policy and Law, Vol. 45, No. 2, April 2020
DOI 10.1215/03616878-8004898   © 2020 by Duke University Press

challenges estimating the scope of the opioid epidemic and the effectiveness of efforts to address opioid use disorder, overdose, and death (Barocas et al. 2018). First responders, communities, and families at the frontlines of the epidemic grapple with ever-evolving terrains and uncertainties over how to promote care, safety, and recovery. These frontline members of the public are crucial actors in efforts to address the opioid epidemic. While knowledge alone cannot solve the opioid epidemic, redressing information asymmetries about opioids features prominently in long-standing justifications for regulatory policy making and for public health information campaigns.

Educating the public through information campaigns constitutes a commonly used policy approach to public health problems. Experimental approaches to assessing the impact of information campaigns, however, may misestimate the effects of such campaigns by failing to account for respondents' willingness to receive new information. Using a survey experiment of a national sample of 1,000 respondents conducted through the YouGov platform, this article examines public willingness to seek new information and update their preferences for health policies related to the opioid epidemic. Is the public receptive to new information on the sources of the opioid epidemic and possible remedies? What are the potential implications of the public's heterogeneity for the development and distribution of health information? We offer some preliminary insight on these puzzles. Notably, among individuals who are likely to receive information, our informational treatment has a large positive effect on increasing support for policies to address the opioid epidemic by about one half of a standard deviation. Among individuals who are likely to avoid this information, policy preferences appear to be unmoved by our treatment. These effects would be missed by standard experimental designs.

Promoting Public Health through Redressing Information Asymmetries

Educating the Public

Promoting public health through public information constitutes an enduring and foundational part of US health policy making at the federal, state, and local levels. Systematic reviews of public health information campaigns find evidence that information campaigns have had a positive impact on public health concerns ranging from tobacco use (National Cancer Institute 2008) to heart disease (Rochella 2002). Such campaigns are more likely to yield durable improvements in public health, however, when they occur in conjunction with commensurate policy changes and local service provision (Wakefield, Loken, and Hornik 2010).

Despite the potential benefits of information campaigns, formidable challenges confront efforts to educate the public on public health and disease prevention. In general, members of the public vary in their likelihood of encountering information (Zaller 1992); and when they do, they may be inclined to discount information that does not comport with their prior predispositions (Kunda 1990) or that comes from sources they deem not credible (Lupia 2013). Without sufficient context, reports of research findings can exacerbate fatalistic beliefs or induce information overload.[2]

These general concerns about the effectiveness of information campaigns manifest in opioid-specific experiments as well. In the context of opioids information and messaging, like other public health challenges, frames and images matter. Referring to the same type of intervention, using the phrase "overdose prevention sites" garnered more public support in experimental conditions than the phrase "safe consumption site" (Barry, Sherman, and McGinty 2018). The images that experiments use to portray opioid addiction also bear on public respondents' support for punitive policies or support for expanded insurance coverage (Kennedy-Hendricks, McGinty, Barry 2016). More broadly, the ways in which public health messages are framed can augment partisan differences in public opinion (Gollust, Lantz, and Ubel 2009). Moreover, correcting inaccurate myths about disease or interventions does not necessarily yield an improvement in behaviors that promote public health (Nyhan and Reifler 2015). These challenges manifest in regulatory agencies' information-based public health strategies as well.

Information, Education, and Regulation of Pharmaceuticals

Information as a policy instrument to influence health behaviors can target individuals directly, and it can pass through intermediaries such as physicians or pharmacists. The FDA, for instance, engages in both direct and indirect public education through postmarketing regulatory communication that comes in several forms including drug labels, medication guides, safety alerts, and warnings. Part of the logic of government-initiated information distribution assumes consumer empowerment: that information

2. These findings focus on the differences that emerge between television and print reports of research findings in the case of cancer (Gollust, Fowler, and Niederdeppe 2019).

will facilitate patients' abilities to engage actively in their pharmaceutical choices, rather than rely solely on physicians as intermediary experts (Grossman 2014). In practice, patients and consumers struggle to understand the pharmaceutical information they receive, leading to frequent calls for clear, simple language when communicating with patients and consumers (Hoek et al. 2011). The effectiveness of these materials depends on consumers reading the label and absorbing the intended message. Yet, studies consistently demonstrate that patients and providers "do not consistently heed [drug] labels" developed to guide and support safe and effective drug use (IOM 2007: 59).[3] When they do take the time to read a warning, they may or may not accurately act in ways consistent with the intent of the warning (Dusetzina et al. 2012). Consumers, for example, may interpret right-to-know disclosures as a strong warning against using the product at all, when the warning was intended to elicit a more moderated consumer response (Bar-Gill, Schkade, and Sunstein 2018).

While some studies find low consumer understanding of drug warnings overall (Ip et al. 2015), others highlight the risks and disadvantage facing consumers with limited English skills (Bailey et al. 2011) or limited health literacy (Yin et al. 2013).[4] Pharmacies do not typically provide drug prescribing and safety information in patients' native languages (Bailey et al. 2011). Despite guidelines calling for the information on drug labels and in medication guides to be written at a 6th–8th grade reading level, medication guides, on average, are written at an 11th–12th grade reading level (Wolf et al. 2006). Moreover, many consumers lack the contextual knowledge needed to understand the words and figures presented in drug information, which makes it difficult or impossible for them to use the information appropriately, even if they successfully read it (Ben-Shahar and Schneider 2014). Low health literacy leads patients to have a harder time understanding medication guides (Wolf et al. 2012; Wolf et al. 2014), to be more likely to misinterpret the risks of a medical procedure (Ben-Shahar and Schneider 2014), or to be more likely take an unsafe dosage of over-the-counter medications (Yin et al. 2013). Uncertainty over the effectiveness of information campaigns also arises because of the piecemeal nature of most studies. Much of what we know about individual-level responses to safety information comes from studies of particular drugs

3. Scholarship on mandated disclosures similarly suggests consumers often skip these warnings (Ben-Shahar and Schneider 2014).

4. Regarding limited English skills, some states, including California and New York, require prescription containers to be translated. Laws do not require the translation of materials such as medication guides (Regenstein et al. 2012).

(Kuehn 2012),[5] yielding uncertainty over whether the findings extend to other disease indications or patient groups.

In the context of the opioid epidemic, the FDA, along with other federal agencies, has deployed a range of information-based policy approaches.[6] These have included the 2003 FDA warning letter on oxycodone, the 2009 FDA education campaign for prescribers and patients, and the 2012 implementation of the Risk Evaluation and Mitigation Strategies for all opioids. Public health advisories have also emerged from the surgeon general, including the recent call for greater access to naloxone.[7] Similarly, many state legislatures have enacted laws mandating the development and inclusion of education about opioids abuse in school curricula.[8]

Empirical Puzzles

Redressing information asymmetries, alone, will not solve the opioid epidemic. Yet efforts to inform the public remain part of the core mission of many agencies and often a key component of more holistic strategies to address this issue. Existing research has demonstrated the broad importance of the framing and content of information about opioids for the general public. Yet broader theories of public opinion imply a more complicated process only partly captured by past work.

Consider two examples using Zaller's (1992) general Receive-Accept-Sample model as a framework to illustrate how the results from an experiment may differ from the dynamics in the world. First, suppose that, as Zaller contends in his reception axiom, exposure to information is correlated with engagement on that issue. In an experiment where information is provided about a complex issue like opioids, the effects of such novel information may be large, since many people are encountering information they have never received before (and are unlikely to otherwise receive

5. For instance, much is known about the effects of warnings associated with antidepressant use (Parkinson et al. 2014; Valluri et al. 2010).

6. The FDA has, of course, also deployed a range of regulatory approaches that go beyond information. The FDA can constrain patients' and providers' access to drugs through restrictions on who can prescribe the drugs, how drug refills can occur, and where refills can occur (GAO 2011: 17).

7. HHS.org, Office of the Surgeon General. "U.S. Surgeon General's Advisory on Naloxone and Opioid Overdose." www.surgeongeneral.gov/priorities/opioid-overdose-prevention/naloxone-advisory.html (accessed January 20, 2019).

8. See the National Conference of State Legislature's "Injury Prevention Legislation Database | Opioid Abuse Prevention" (www.ncsl.org/research/health/injury-prevention-legislation-database .aspx; accessed June 15, 2019) for a searchable database. For example, in 2017, Pennsylvania passed HB 178, which directs the state's Department of Health and Department of Drug and Alcohol Programs to develop a model curriculum on the issue.

in the course of their daily lives). Yet among the small subset of those engaged with the issue—people who care about opioids and follow the issue closely—the effects may be small or nonexistent, as they already know the information being provided. Second, suppose exposure is correlated with prior beliefs. People likely to encounter the information respond as one would hope, becoming more informed and supportive of particular policy, while people who would choose to avoid this information resist the information provided because it conflicts with their prior beliefs, and they move their opinions in the opposite direction of the treatment's desired effects (Zaller's 1992 resistance axiom). Depending on the size of these two groups, the effects we observe in an experiment might be close to zero, leading us to conclude a campaign is ineffective when the campaign has the desired effect among the population it is likely to reach. Rather than try to infer these processes through measures like education or knowledge that may proxy for exposure and measures like partisanship or ideology that may proxy for resistance, we detail in the next section how scholars can learn more by trying to directly incorporate these dynamics into the design and analysis of their studies.

Data and Design

When will the public seek out information on opioids and what consequence will that information have? Standard survey experiments provide only a partial answer to these questions, offering an estimate of the effect of treatment when everyone receives it (Gaines, Kuklinski, and Quirk 2007). Instead, scholars and policy makers may wish to know the effects of some informational campaign on those likely to receive it. They may also wish to know how such messages will be received by audiences unlikely to be exposed to such information as divergent responses may suggest the need for alternative communication strategies.

We explore these questions through an experimental design in which some subjects are given an opportunity to choose whether to receive information about opioid abuse in the US, while others are randomly assigned exposure to these facts: information that they may or may not have otherwise chosen to avoid. Experimental designs of this type are common in public health, where they are generally known as patient preference trials (Long, Little, and Lin 2008; Rücker 1989; Torgersen, Klaber-Moffett, and Russell 1996). They have been used in political science to assess the effects of negative campaigns and partisan media (Arceneaux, Johnson, and Murphy 2012; Gaines, Kuklinski and Quirk 2007; Knox et al. 2019).

Before asking you more about your views on opioid abuse in the U.S., we'd like to share with you some facts about this issue:

- Every **12 minutes**, someone in America **dies** from a prescription or illicit opioid overdose
- In 2016, **1 in 5 deaths** among **young adults** were opioid related.
- Heroin–related overdose deaths were **five times higher** in 2016 compared to 2010.
- **80% heroin** users started with a **prescription painkiller**.
- In 2016, enough painkillers were prescribed by healthcare providers to medicate **every American adult** with 30mg hydrocodone **everyday for almost a month**

Figure 1 Informational treatment seen by respondents who were either randomly assigned or elected to hear more information about the opioid crisis.

Our particular study employs a parallel design in which some subjects are randomly assigned to treatment while other subjects are given the choice of whether to receive treatment or not. Subjects were asked two questions about opioid abuse in the US: whether they personally knew someone who had been addicted to prescription painkillers or other opioids and for an assessment of the extent to which opioid abuse was a major problem in the area in which they live. Subjects were then randomly assigned to one of two experimental conditions. Approximately 30% of subjects were assigned to a simple experimental design in which they were randomly assigned to treatment or control with equal probability. Treated subjects were presented with a brief set of informational facts (figure 1) about the opioid crisis taken from an information project by the Truth Initiative, a nonprofit organization,[9] before answering a set of outcome measures detailed below. The treatment aims to mimic the kind of information presented in public health campaigns and often cited in media coverage of the opioid epidemic. Subjects in the control proceed directly to the questions.

The remaining 70% of subjects were assigned to a selection experiment in which they were given the option, shown in figure 2, of whether to read some more information on the issue before providing their own on the views on the issue.

Subjects who responded "yes" received the information presented in figure 1. Subjects who responded "no" proceeded directly to our battery of outcome measures. For subjects who received the informational treatment, the survey paused for 5 seconds before respondents could advance to the next section.

Figure 3 provides a summary of our experimental design and helps illustrate two key strengths of parallel design. First, as the right-hand side

9. See "Get the Facts" (www.thetruth.com/the-facts; accessed October 15, 2018).

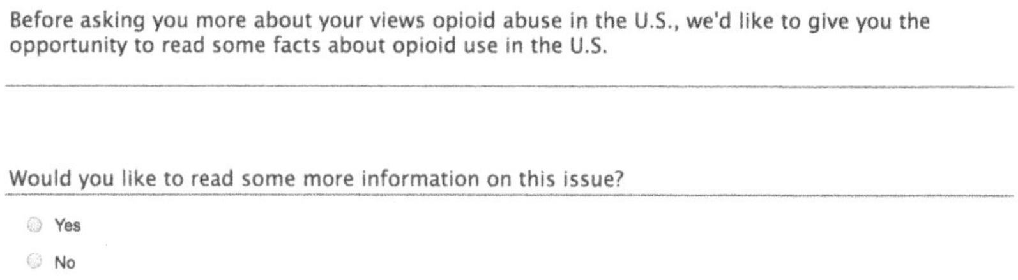

Before asking you more about your views opioid abuse in the U.S., we'd like to give you the opportunity to read some facts about opioid use in the U.S.

Would you like to read some more information on this issue?

   ○ Yes

   ○ No

Figure 2 Informational choice provided to the subjects in the selection condition of the experiment.

of the figure shows, we can represent the average treatment effect from a standard survey experiment ($E[Y|D=T]-E[Y|D=C]$) as the weighted average of the treatment effects among those likely to seek out information τ_s and those likely to avoid such information τ_a. Second, as the left-hand side of figure 3 shows, we can estimate the proportion α of the people likely to seek out information on opioids when given the chance. With these quantities we can estimate what Knox et al. (2019) refer to as the Average Choice-Specific Treatment Effects (ACTEs) by taking the difference between the average outcome in the selection condition, (that is, the weighted average of those who selected both into and out of treatment, $E[Y|C=C]$), and the average of those in the control (in this study, those randomly assigned to read the treatment, $E[Y|C=E, D=C]$), and weighting this estimate by the proportion of people likely to select that treatment:

$$ACTE_{\text{Select}} = \frac{\overbrace{[E[Y|C=C]}^{\text{Average: Choice}} - \overbrace{E[Y|C=E,D=C]}^{\text{Average: Control}}}{\underbrace{\alpha}_{\text{Proportion Selecting Treatment}}} \quad \bullet$$

Similarly, we can recover the effect of treatment on those likely to avoid it (τ_a) by taking the difference between the average outcome among those assigned to treatment, $E[Y|C=E, D=T]$, and the average outcome among those allowed to select into or out of treatment, $E[Y|C=C]$, and weighting this difference by the proportion of those likely to avoid that treatment $(1-\alpha)$.

$$ACTE_{\text{Avoid}} = \frac{\overbrace{[E[Y|C=E,D=T]}^{\text{Average: Treatment}} - \overbrace{E[Y|C=C]}^{\text{Average: Choice}}}{\underbrace{(1-\alpha)}_{\text{Proportion Avoiding Treatment}}}$$

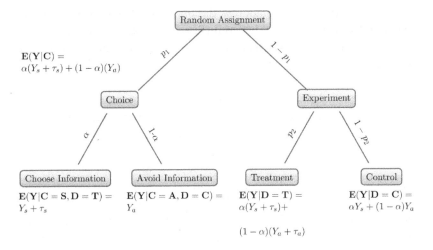

Figure 3   Doubly randomized parallel design.

Standard errors for a ratio of estimates can be constructed via the delta method (Cameron and Trivedi 2005).

Data, Outcomes, and Measurement

The data for our study come from a larger survey of 1,000 respondents conducted by the Taubman Center for American Politics and Policy in the fall of 2018 and fielded by polling firm YouGov. YouGov uses matched sampling with poststratification weights to obtain a nationally representative sample from its online panel (Rivers 2006). The median respondent in our sample was a 47-year-old white woman with some college experience who identifies as being ideologically moderate and a political independent.

We consider three sets of outcomes designed to measure whether our treatment changed respondents' (1) objective knowledge about the opioid crisis, (2) beliefs about the primary cause of this crisis, and (3) support for general policy measures to address this issue. We measure factual knowledge with a binary indicator for whether subjects could correctly recall the percentage of heroin users who started with a prescription painkiller. To assess subjects' beliefs about the causes of the opioid crisis, we use two binary indicators capturing whether subjects believe the primary cause of the present situation is health care providers or illicit drug use. To capture policy preferences, we use a battery of seven items measuring agreement with various approaches to address the opioid epidemic through education, training, regulation, and the criminal justice system on a 7-point scale (1 = strongly disagree, 7 = strongly agree). For simplicity of discussion, we produce two scales from these seven items using principal components analysis to capture general support for more punitive and more treatment-oriented approaches to the opioid crisis. We use standard measures of demographic (age, income, education, gender, and race) and political variables (partisanship and ideology) to describe who is likely to seek out or avoid information and to estimate heterogeneous effects by subgroup to compare our estimates of the overall average treatment effects (ATE) and choice-specific ACTEs. Our survey also contains information on where subjects report receiving information about opioids, and how the opioid crisis makes them feel. These questions, however, were asked posttreatment, and we use them primarily for descriptive and exploratory purposes.

Results

We begin our discussion with a descriptive analysis of where people report receiving information about opioid addiction. Next, we examine the characteristics of who, when given the opportunity to receive more information about this crisis, chooses to receive or avoid that information. Then, we assess the effects of that information, looking first at whether this information increases objective knowledge about the crisis and then whether such information alters what people believe is the primary cause for this crisis and their beliefs about policies to address this crisis. Finally, we explore some possible explanations for why the effects of information appear to differ by the likelihood of receiving it.

Where Do People Get Information about Opioids?

Table 1 presents some descriptive statistics of the self-reported frequency with which people encounter information about opioid addiction from various sources.[10] We see that the news media is far and away the most frequent source of information about opioid addiction with 40% of respondents reporting they frequently received information from the media and another 32% reporting receiving information from this source more infrequently. About half of all respondents report receiving at least some

10. These informational questions were asked posttreatment, and percentages were calculated with responses for subjects in the control condition only (N = 143). Results are unchanged in terms of relative rankings using the full sample of respondents.

Table 1   Sources of Information about Opioid Addiction

	Never	Once or twice	Frequently
Government agencies	57%	33%	10%
Healthcare professionals	50%	38%	12%
Local schools	73%	21%	6%
Family and friends	64%	21%	15%
Pharmaceutical companies	78%	17%	5%
News media	28%	32%	40%

information from health care professionals, 43% report they received information from government agencies, and just over a third report having received information from family and friends. Local schools and pharmaceutical companies were less common sources of information for about a quarter of respondents. Overall, only about 20% of respondents reported receiving no information from any of the six sources, 9% of respondents reported receiving at least some information from all six sources, and nearly two-thirds of respondents reported receiving information from more than one source.

Who Seeks Out Information about the Opioid Crisis?

The results from the previous section suggest a number of policy-relevant patterns about the public's likelihood of encountering information on the opioid crisis. First, a significant portion of the public, about 1 in 5, reports receiving no information from any of the six sources we listed. Second, the remainder of our sample reports receiving information from a relatively diverse array of sources, with the media being the primary and most frequent source of information. We now consider characteristics of who is likely to seek out such information, when given the choice (albeit in the context of taking an online survey) to seek out additional information on the opioid crisis.

Of the 712 subjects assigned to the choice condition in our experiment, 395 elected to receive more information about the opioid crisis (55%), while 317 chose not to receive this information (45%). Figure 4 examines how these two groups of respondents differ along eight dimensions. Subjects who chose to receive additional information were about 8% more likely to report knowing someone who had struggled with addiction (46% vs. 38%, $p < 0.05$) and marginally more likely to report that opioid addiction was a major problem in their community (41% vs. 35%, ns) compared to subjects who opted not to view the additional information.

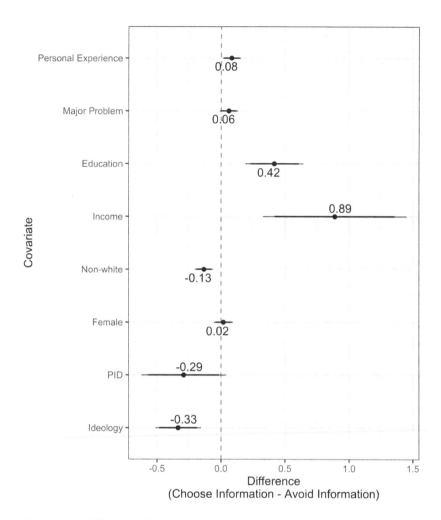

Figure 4 Differences between subjects who choose or avoid additional information on the opioid crisis.

People who elected to receive additional information were also more likely to have higher levels of education and income, less likely to be racial minorities, and more likely to identify as Democrats and liberals.

Effects of Information

The results from figure 4 suggest that people open to receiving information about the opioid crisis differ in a number of ways from those who,

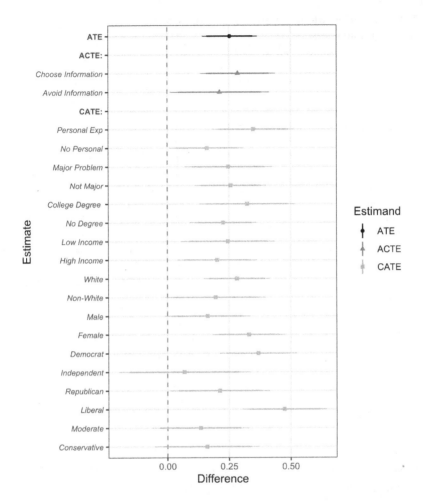

Figure 5 Effect of treatment on factual knowledge of the opioid crisis.

given the choice, might opt to avoid such information. It seems likely, then, that the effects of such information will vary conditional on the likelihood of receiving it.

We examine this possibility first with regard to the objective knowledge subjects gained from our experiment. Figure 5 shows the average treatment effect (ATE) in green, compared to average choice-specific treatment effects (ACTEs) among those likely to choose or avoid our informational

Table 2 Effect of Treatment on Factual Knowledge of the Opioid Crisis

Estimate	Difference	SE	ll	ul	Pr(<|t|)
ATE	0.25	0.06	0.14	0.36	0.00
ACTEs:					
Choose information	0.29	0.08	0.13	0.44	0.00
Avoid information	0.21	0.10	0.01	0.41	0.04
CATEs:					
Personal experience	0.35	0.08	0.18	0.52	0.00
No personal experience	0.16	0.08	0.01	0.31	0.04
Major problem	0.25	0.09	0.07	0.43	0.01
Not major	0.26	0.07	0.11	0.40	0.00
College degree	0.32	0.10	0.13	0.52	0.00
No degree	0.23	0.07	0.09	0.36	0.00
Low income	0.25	0.10	0.06	0.44	0.01
High income	0.20	0.08	0.04	0.36	0.01
White	0.28	0.07	0.15	0.42	0.00
Nonwhite	0.19	0.10	−0.01	0.40	0.06
Male	0.16	0.09	−0.01	0.34	0.07
Female	0.33	0.07	0.18	0.48	0.00
Democrat	0.37	0.08	0.21	0.52	0.00
Independent	0.07	0.13	−0.20	0.33	0.61
Republican	0.21	0.10	0.01	0.41	0.04
Liberal	0.47	0.09	0.30	0.65	0.00
Moderate	0.13	0.10	−0.06	0.33	0.18
Conservative	0.16	0.11	−0.05	0.37	0.14

treatment in red, as well as conditional average treatment effects (CATEs) in blue for the subgroups from the previous section. Point estimates, confidence intervals, and p-values are provided in table 2. Overall, the treatment appeared to increase the probability that respondents would correctly identify the percent of heroin users who started with prescription pain killers by 25 percentage points from 30% in the control 55% in treatment (p < 0.05). The effects are slightly larger for those likely to seek out this information (29 percentage points) compared to those who would avoid this information (21 percentage points), but the differences are nonsignificant. The effects are generally similar in size and sign across various subgroups, ranging from a minimum, nonsignificant increase of 6 percentage points for independents and a maximum increase of 47 percentage points among liberals (p < 0.05).

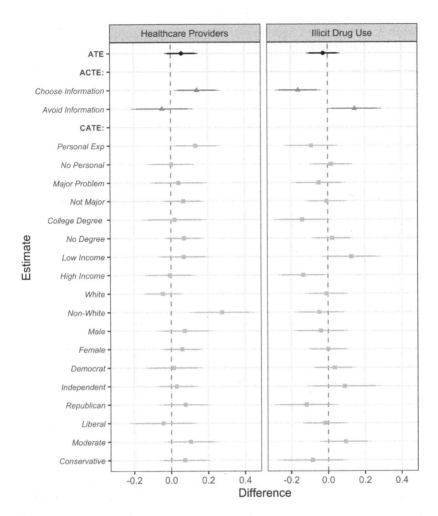

Figure 6   Effect of treatment on beliefs about the primary cause of the opioid crisis.

These initial results provide evidence that people did in fact receive and understand the treatment. But it should not be too surprising that when you provide people with simple, factual information many of them are able to recall this information when prompted shortly thereafter. The more interesting question is what people do with this information and how they update their beliefs and preferences.

Figure 6 examines the effects of treatment on subjects' beliefs about the primary cause of the opioid crisis—specifically, the extent to which

Table 3 Treatment Effect on Attributing Opioid Crisis
to Health Care Providers

Estimate	Difference	SE	ll	ul	Pr(<|t|)
ATE	0.06	0.05	−0.03	0.15	0.20
ACTEs:					
Choose information	0.14	0.06	0.02	0.27	0.02
Avoid information	−0.05	0.09	−0.21	0.12	0.59
CATEs:					
Personal experience	0.14	0.07	0.00	0.27	0.05
No personal experience	0.00	0.06	−0.12	0.13	0.96
Major problem	0.04	0.08	−0.11	0.20	0.59
Not major	0.07	0.06	−0.04	0.18	0.23
College degree	0.02	0.09	−0.15	0.20	0.81
No degree	0.07	0.05	−0.04	0.18	0.19
Low income	0.07	0.07	−0.07	0.21	0.32
High income	−0.01	0.07	−0.14	0.13	0.94
White	−0.05	0.05	−0.15	0.05	0.37
Nonwhite	0.28	0.09	0.10	0.45	0.00
Male	0.07	0.08	−0.08	0.22	0.33
Female	0.06	0.06	−0.05	0.17	0.30
Democrat	0.01	0.08	−0.14	0.17	0.86
Independent	0.03	0.06	−0.08	0.14	0.59
Republican	0.08	0.07	−0.07	0.22	0.29
Liberal	−0.04	0.09	−0.23	0.14	0.63
Moderate	0.10	0.07	−0.04	0.25	0.16
Conservative	0.07	0.07	−0.06	0.21	0.28

subjects are likely to attribute responsibility for the present crisis to health
care providers (left-hand panel) or illicit drug use (right-hand panel).
Point estimates, confidence intervals, and p-values are provided in tables 3
and 4. Three features of these results are particularly striking. First, in
both cases, a standard survey experiment would suggest that our informational treatment had no effect. Second, these null results for the ATE
mask significant substantive differences uncovered by our ability to estimate ACTEs for people likely and unlikely to receive our treatment.
Specifically, subjects who would opt to receive information when given
the chance are more likely to attribute blame to health care providers
and less likely to attribute blame for the current crisis to illicit drug use.
In contrast, when subjects who would prefer not to receive any additional
information about the opioid crisis do receive that information, they are

Table 4   Treatment Effect on Attributing Opioid Crisis
to Illicit Drug Use

Estimate	Difference	SE	ll	ul	Pr(<|t|)
ATE	−0.02	0.05	−0.11	0.07	0.60
ACTEs:					
Choose information	−0.16	0.06	−0.28	−0.04	0.01
Avoid information	0.15	0.08	−0.00	0.29	0.05
CATEs:					
Personal experience	−0.09	0.07	−0.24	0.06	0.23
No personal experience	0.02	0.06	−0.10	0.13	0.77
Major problem	−0.05	0.07	−0.20	0.10	0.51
Not major	−0.01	0.06	−0.12	0.11	0.91
College degree	−0.14	0.08	−0.29	0.01	0.07
No degree	0.02	0.06	−0.09	0.13	0.70
Low income	0.13	0.08	−0.03	0.29	0.12
High income	−0.13	0.07	−0.27	0.00	0.05
White	−0.01	0.06	−0.12	0.11	0.89
Nonwhite	−0.05	0.07	−0.18	0.09	0.48
Male	−0.04	0.07	−0.19	0.11	0.60
Female	−0.00	0.06	−0.11	0.11	0.99
Democrat	0.03	0.06	−0.08	0.15	0.56
Independent	0.09	0.10	−0.12	0.29	0.39
Republican	−0.12	0.09	−0.29	0.06	0.18
Liberal	−0.02	0.06	−0.14	0.11	0.78
Moderate	0.09	0.07	−0.05	0.23	0.19
Conservative	−0.08	0.10	−0.28	0.11	0.38

no more likely to blame health care providers and in fact are about 15 percentage points more likely to say the current crisis is caused primarily by illicit drug use (p < 0.05). Third, standard subgroup analysis is unlikely to detect this heterogeneity as most of the CATEs are nonsignificant; and no clear pattern emerges across the few estimates that are significant. For example, why should personal experience and race condition attributions about health care providers but not about illicit drug use? Or, why should ideology and partisanship, significant predictors of subgroup heterogeneity in the previous section, not predict more variation here? Instead, by incorporating the dynamics of choice directly into the design and analysis of experiment, we have uncovered effects that we might have otherwise missed.

Next, we examine the extent to which our brief informational treatment influenced subjects' general support for policies to address the opioid

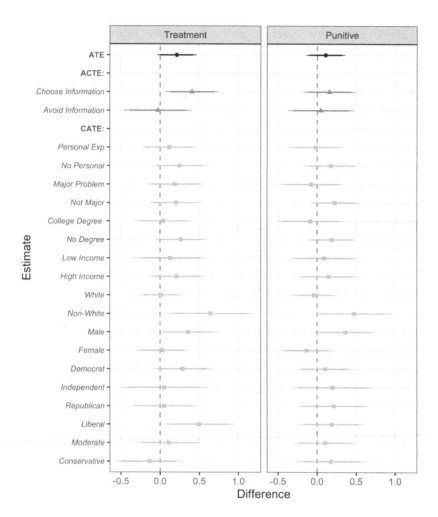

Figure 7 Effect of treatment on support for policy responses to the opioid crisis.

crisis through more treatment-focused approaches emphasizing education, regulation, and health care, and more punitive approaches emphasizing arresting dealers and users. Figure 7 presents the ATE, ACTEs, and CATEs from our analysis using our summary measures of policy beliefs (point estimates, confidence intervals, and p-values in tables 5 and 6). Again, we see a similar pattern of results to what we found when considering causal attributions.

Table 5 Treatment Effects on Support for More Treatment-Oriented Policies

Estimate	Difference	SE	ll	ul	Pr(<|t|)
ATE	0.21	0.13	−0.04	0.46	0.10
ACTEs:					
Choose information	0.40	0.17	0.06	0.74	0.02
Avoid information	−0.03	0.22	−0.46	0.40	0.89
CATEs:					
Personal experience	0.12	0.18	−0.23	0.47	0.51
No personal experience	0.24	0.18	−0.10	0.59	0.16
Major problem	0.19	0.18	−0.17	0.55	0.30
Not major	0.20	0.17	−0.13	0.54	0.22
College degree	0.04	0.19	−0.33	0.42	0.83
No degree	0.27	0.16	−0.05	0.58	0.10
Low income	0.13	0.23	−0.33	0.59	0.58
High income	0.21	0.17	−0.14	0.56	0.23
White	0.01	0.13	−0.26	0.27	0.96
Nonwhite	0.64	0.28	0.08	1.20	0.02
Male	0.36	0.19	−0.02	0.73	0.06
Female	0.03	0.16	−0.30	0.35	0.87
Democrat	0.29	0.19	−0.09	0.66	0.13
Independent	0.05	0.28	−0.50	0.60	0.85
Republican	0.05	0.21	−0.36	0.46	0.81
Liberal	0.50	0.22	0.05	0.94	0.03
Moderate	0.11	0.21	−0.30	0.52	0.60
Conservative	−0.14	0.21	−0.56	0.28	0.51

Among those likely to receive this information, treatment has a large positive effect on increasing support for treatment-oriented policies to address the opioid epidemic but no effect on support for more punitive approaches. Among those who would avoid this information, preferences appear to be unmoved by treatment. These effects would be missed if we looked only at the ATE from our experiment, and analysis of subgroups yields some idiosyncratic evidence of heterogeneity.

As noted above, people who chose to receive information about the opioid crisis differed in a number of observable ways from those who elected to avoid such information, but those differences fail to predictably explain the divergent pattern of responses we see among those likely and unlikely to receive our treatment. We conclude with a brief, exploratory analysis of some of the ways these two groups—information seekers and avoiders—differ in their emotional evaluations of the opioid crisis. While

Table 6 Treatment Effects on Support for More Punitive Policies

Estimate	Difference	SE	ll	ul	Pr(<|t|)
ATE	0.11	0.13	−0.14	0.35	0.39
ACTEs:					
Choose information	0.16	0.17	−0.18	0.49	0.36
Avoid information	0.05	0.22	−0.38	0.47	0.83
CATEs:					
Personal experience	−0.02	0.18	−0.37	0.33	0.92
No personal experience	0.17	0.18	−0.18	0.52	0.33
Major problem	−0.07	0.21	−0.48	0.33	0.72
Not major	0.23	0.15	−0.08	0.53	0.14
College degree	−0.09	0.21	−0.51	0.34	0.69
No degree	0.19	0.15	−0.12	0.49	0.23
Low income	0.09	0.21	−0.34	0.51	0.68
High income	0.15	0.19	−0.23	0.52	0.44
White	−0.05	0.14	−0.33	0.24	0.75
Nonwhite	0.47	0.25	−0.02	0.96	0.06
Male	0.36	0.19	−0.02	0.75	0.07
Female	−0.13	0.16	−0.45	0.18	0.40
Democrat	0.10	0.18	−0.25	0.46	0.56
Independent	0.20	0.26	−0.33	0.72	0.45
Republican	0.21	0.22	−0.23	0.65	0.34
Liberal	0.19	0.21	−0.23	0.60	0.38
Moderate	0.10	0.20	−0.29	0.50	0.60
Conservative	0.18	0.22	−0.27	0.62	0.43

primarily a descriptive exercise, it may help explain why, when presented with the same information, people seem to respond in divergent manners. Figure 8 presents the average responses across each of our four treatment groups to a set of questions asking subjects how often they felt angry, empathetic, indifferent, powerless, resentful, and sad toward individuals addicted to opioids. In no case did our brief informational treatment appear to influence subjects' summary emotional evaluations of this larger issue. But as the bottom set of averages illustrate, people willing to seek out information on the opioid crisis feel very differently toward those addicted to opioids than those who would avoid such information do. Those open to receiving information are less likely to report feeling indifferent and resentful and more likely to report feeling empathetic, powerless, and sad. As an early exploratory exercise, these descriptive results may help shed light on why information effects these two groups differently.

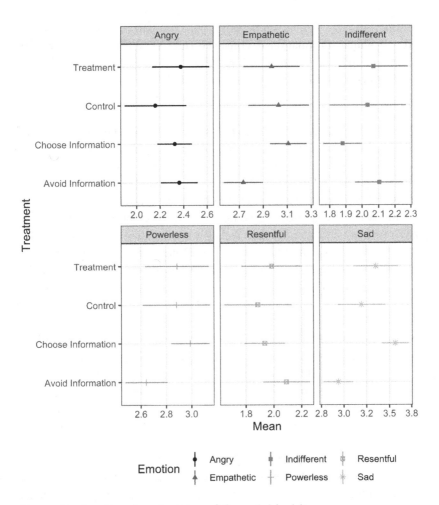

Figure 8 Emotional evaluations of the opioid crisis.

Limitations, Alternative Explanations, and Future Research

In this section we consider some possible threats to the validity of our inferences as well as some alternative explanations for our reported results. First, while we believe our approach possesses greater external validity than standard forced-exposure designs common to other experimental studies, it is hard, if not impossible, to perfectly capture the informational choices of everyday life. Alternative designs might vary the type of information (e.g., factual statistics vs. personal narratives) or the format through which information is conveyed (text vs. audio), as well as the number of choices presented although increasing the diversity of choices requires imposing additional assumptions and analytical constraints (see Knox et al. 2019). While the present experiment may not perfectly capture real life (few if any do), we believe it provides a reasonable approximation of the kind of choices people make when deciding whether to read an article or throw out an informational postcard. Another fruitful direction for further research would be to examine the dynamics of choice over time (Broockman and Kalla 2016; Druckman, Fein, and Leeper 2012).

Second, a threat to the internal validity of our estimates arises from the possibility that when offered the choice to read information, people process that information differently than if they'd been randomly assigned to that information (Evans and Stanovich 2013; Kahneman 2011). For example, dual-process models of human cognition posit two systems for how individuals process information. System 1 captures the automatic processes like heuristics that individuals use to process information efficiently, while system 2 describes the more active, deliberate thinking individuals engage in when presented with a task that requires cognitive effort. It is possible, then, that most subjects in the experimental arm of the survey are engaged in the default of system 1 processing, while subjects given a choice are prompted to engage in more effortful, system 2 processing. A related concern comes from the possibility that our choice condition creates demand effects, where respondents are adjusting their responses to match the presumed desired responses of researchers (Orne 1962).

While these are important and valid concerns, we believe our main results still hold for the following reasons. First, with regard to demand effects, Mummolo and Peterson (2019) suggest online survey experiments may be less affected by such concerns and present evidence showing little difference in treatment effects even when subjects are provided with information and incentives related to an experiment's purpose (see also de Quidt, Haushofer, and Roth 2018). Second, if our study is subject to demand effects, it seems unlikely that the bias would be particularly larger among subjects given the choice to receive information compared to subjects randomly assigned to receive it. And indeed, for our measure of factual knowledge, the ATE and ACTEs are quite similar.

Where these estimates diverge, it is possible that these differences reflect a pattern of systematically different cognitive processing induced by our experimental treatment; but, again, we believe several factors weigh against this interpretation as the sole explanation for our results. First, for all subjects who received the information, the survey paused for a brief period (5 seconds) to ensure that subjects had time to read the facts. Second, the total survey times for respondents who selected to read the article where not statistically distinguishable from those randomly assigned to read the article. Third, we believe the descriptive differences in emotional evaluations of the opioid crisis by decision to encounter information are more consistent with persistent differences in how people process that information rather than design-induced changes in the way people cognitively processed our informational treatment. Still, we cannot rule out this interpretation— and future studies using similar designs might explicitly include measures designed to distinguish between attitude changes arising from system 1 versus system 2 processing.

Finally, we have broadly argued that our results show how the effects of information about the opioid crisis vary based on the likelihood that a person encounters it. For policy makers, we believe the effect of some intervention on its likely recipients is often of particular interest. Of course, policy makers and scholars may also wish to know why a treatment had the effect it did and why that effect varied. Here too, we believe our design offers added insights above standard approaches. As figure 4 shows, people opting into and out of our informational treatment differ along a number of theoretically relevant dimensions—people who received the information were more likely to have personal experience with the opioid crisis, to have higher levels of income and education, more likely to be white, and to be more Democratic and liberal. In further exploratory analysis conditioning on these subgroups, we find a similar pattern of effects to the main results among those without a college degree, but generally no effect among those with a 2-year degree or higher. With regard to partisanship, we find some suggestive and surprising patterns. For example, independents who would choose to receive information are more likely to attribute blame for the opioid crisis to health care providers, while independents who would avoid information are less likely to do so. Our claim is not that these factors don't matter, but instead that many of them are likely to matter in ways that condition both exposure and response to information. By allowing researchers to observe this process directly, our design creates opportunities and insights for future research to explore why one message worked the way it did or how a different message might be tailored to reach a particular audience in the context of the opioid crisis specifically or in the context of other public information campaigns more broadly.

Conclusion

Having a better-informed public is a foundational component of public health in the US. Yet, how to inform the public effectively remains elusive. Our parallel design, in which some subjects are randomly assigned to treatment while other subjects are given the choice of whether to receive treatment or not, offers a window into the public's heterogeneity that could benefit future information-focused efforts related to opioids. While our experimental intervention increased basic knowledge of the opioid crisis among all respondents, how that information shaped respondents' beliefs varied by how likely they were to encounter it. Among those likely to receive information, treatment altered attributions of blame for the opioid crisis, decreasing the likelihood of attributing the crisis to the behavior of users and increasing the likelihood of attributing the crisis to the behavior of health care providers. Respondents who were open to receiving this message were more supportive of treatment-oriented policies to address the opioid epidemic by about one half of a standard deviation. Among those who would avoid this information, policy preferences appear to be unmoved by treatment; and encountering this information increased the probability of blaming drug users for the current crisis. While redressing information asymmetries is only one part of a public health strategy for addressing the opioid epidemic, our findings highlight the importance of access to and receptiveness toward new information.

Recognizing that mitigating the current epidemic will require a wide range of interventions, our results highlight important terrain for future research.[11] For one, the current structure of FDA impact analyses insufficiently considers the downstream effects of its information-based regulatory interventions. By that, we mean that the FDA does not sufficiently analyze whether the ways in which it reports information to the public—through labels, medication guides, advisories—will reach different kinds of patient groups (including differences by socioeconomic status, health literacy, English proficiency, and gender, among others). Nor does the agency assess potential disparate effects of those information campaigns on different groups. Future research could analyze whether there are ways government agencies' information-based efforts could incorporate the public's heterogeneity more fully into information designs and what effects that might have on information access and use.

For another, has the opioid epidemic damaged public trust in health care providers as credible sources of information? And, if so, what are the

---

11. On the range of community-based interventions for managing the epidemic, see Fraser and Plescia 2019.

implications of this damage for future efforts to convey important information to the public via health care professionals? Recent surveys suggest "the public placed the most blame on doctors who inappropriately prescribe painkillers" when asked "who is mainly responsible for the growing [opioid] problem" (Blendon and Benson 2018). Given the importance of receiving information from credible sources, future research should examine who the public—or different subpopulations of the public—deem credible.

In the words of one former FDA director, drug safety and effectiveness "is a complex problem that is not solved by government, not solved by FDA alone, and not solved for just one drug" (FDA 2000). Information asymmetries are only one part of the complex set of reasons that the opioid epidemic emerged. Redressing information asymmetries will be only one part of mitigating the crisis. But, even within the narrow sphere of informational approaches, the results of our experiments highlight the complexity of understanding the effects of information.

■ ■ ■

Paul F. Testa is an assistant professor in the Department of Political Science at Brown University. His research focuses on how interactions with the criminal justice system shape political behavior. His work has appeared in *American Journal of Political Science, Journal of Oncology Practice, Political Behavior,* and *Public Research Quarterly.* He is an affiliate with the Taubman Center for American Politics and Policy and an advisor to the Policy Lab at Brown University.
paul_testa@brown.edu

Susan L. Moffitt is the director of the Taubman Center for American Politics and Policy and an associate professor in the Department of Political Science at Brown University. Her research focuses on putting policy into practice in the fields of public education and public health. Her publications include two books: *Making Policy Public: Participatory Bureaucracy in American Democracy* (2014) and *The Ordeal of Equality: Did Federal Regulation Fix the Schools* (2009), coauthored with David K. Cohen. Before joining the faculty at Brown University, she was a Robert Wood Johnson Scholar in health policy research at Harvard University.

Marie Schenk is a PhD candidate in the Department of Political Science at Brown University. Her research focuses on how everyday political discussions shape political identity and civic engagement, with a particular interest in the use of big data and experimental methods.

Acknowledgments

We are grateful to the Taubman Center for American Politics and Policy for including our survey experiment on the 2019 fall YouGov survey.

References

Arceneaux, Kevin, Martin Johnson, and Chad Murphy. 2012. "Polarized Political Communication, Oppositional Media Hostility, and Selective Exposure." *Journal of Politics* 74, no. 1: 174–86.

Bailey, Stacy Cooper, Nisha Agarwal, Betsy Sleath, Serena Gumusoglu, and Michael S. Wolf. 2011. "Improving Drug Labeling and Counseling for Limited English Proficient Adults." *Journal of Health Care for the Poor and Underserved* 22, no. 4: 1131–43.

Bar-Gill, Oren, David Schkade, and Cass R. Sunstein. 2018. "Drawing False Inferences from Mandated Disclosures." *Behavioural Public Policy* 3, no. 2: 209–27. doi.org/10.1017/bpp.2017.12.

Barocas, Joshua A., Laura F. White, Jianing Wang, Alexander Y. Walley, Marc R. LaRochelle, Dana Bernson, Thomas Land, Jake R. Morgan, Jeffrey H. Samet, and Benjamin P. Linas. 2018. "Estimated Prevalence of Opioid Use Disorder in Massachusetts, 2011–2015: A Capture–Recapture Analysis." *American Journal of Public Health* 108, no. 12: 1675–81.

Barry, Colleen L., Susan G. Sherman, and Emma E. McGinty. 2018. "Language Matters in Combatting the Opioid Epidemic: Safe Consumption Sites versus Overdose Prevention Sites." *American Journal of Public Health* 108, no. 9: 1157–59.

Ben-Shahar, Omri, and Carl E. Schneider. 2014. *More Than You Wanted to Know: The Failure of Mandated Disclosure*. Princeton, NJ: Princeton University Press.

Blendon, Robert J., and John M. Benson. 2018. "The Public and the Opioid-Abuse Epidemic." *New England Journal of Medicine* 378, no. 5: 407–11.

Bonnie, Richard, Mark A. Schumacher, J. David Clark, and Aaron S. Kesselheim. 2019. "Pain Management and Opioid Regulation: Continuing Public Health Challenges." *American Journal of Public Health* 109, no. 1: 31–34.

Broockman, David, and Joshua Kalla. 2016. "Durably Reducing Transphobia: A Field Experiment on Door-to-Door Canvassing." *Science* 352, no. 6282: 220–24.

Cameron, A. Colin, and Pravin K. Trivedi. 2005. *Microeconometrics: Methods and Applications*. Cambridge: Cambridge University Press.

de Quidt, Jonathan, Johannes Haushofer, and Christopher Roth. 2018. "Measuring and Bounding Experimenter Demand." *American Economic Review* 108, no. 11: 3266–302.

Druckman, James N., Jordan Fein, and Thomas J. Leeper. 2012. "A Source of Bias in Public Opinion Stability." *American Political Science Review* 106, no. 2: 430–54.

Dusetzina, Stacie B., Ashley S. Higashi, E. Ray Dorsey, Rena Conti, Haiden A. Huskamp, Shu Zhu, Craif F. Garfield, and G. Caleb Alexander. 2012. "Impact of

FDA Drug Risk Communications on Health Care Utilization and Health Behaviors." *Medical Care* 50, no. 6: 466–78.

Evans, Jonathan St. B. T., and Keith E. Stanovich. 2013. "Dual-Process Theories of Higher Cognition: Advancing the Debate." *Perspectives on Psychological Science* 8, no. 3: 223–41.

FDA (Food and Drug Administration). 2000. "Gastrointestinal Drugs Advisory Committee Meeting Transcript: Lotronex." June 27. wayback.archive-it.org /7993/20170403222328/https://www.fda.gov/ohrms/dockets/ac/cder00.htm# Gastrointestinal.

Fraser, Michael, and Marcus Plescia. 2019. "The Opioid Epidemic's Prevention Problem." *American Journal of Public Health* 109, no. 2: 215–17.

Gaines, Brian J., James H. Kuklinski, and Paul J. Quirk. 2007. "The Logic of the Survey Experiment Reexamined." *Political Analysis* 15, no. 1: 1–20.

GAO (US Government Accountability Office). 2011. *Prescription Pain Reliever Abuse: Agencies Have Begun Coordinating Efforts, but Need to Assess Effectiveness.* GAO 12–115. Washington, DC: US Government Accountability Office.

Gollust, Sarah E., Erika Franklin Fowler, and Jeff Niederdeppe. 2019. "Television News Coverage of Public Health Issues and Implications for Public Health Policy and Practice." *Annual Review of Public Health* 40, no. 1: 167–85.

Gollust, Sarah E., Paula M. Lantz, and Peter A. Ubel. 2009. "The Polarizing Effect of News Media on the Social Determinants of Health." *American Journal of Public Health* 99, no. 12: 2160–67.

Grossman, Lewis A. 2014. "FDA and the Rise of the Empowered Consumer." *Administrative Law Review* 66: 627–76.

Hadland, Scott E., Ariadne Rivera-Aguirre, Brandon D. L. Marshall, and Magdalena Cerda. 2019. "Association of Pharmaceutical Industry Marketing of Opioid Products with Mortality from Opioid-Related Overdoses." *JAMA Open* 2, no. 1: e16007.

Hoek, Janet, Philip Gendall, Lara Rapson, and Jordan Louviere. 2011. "Information Accessibility and Consumers' Knowledge of Prescription Drug Benefits and Risks." *Journal of Consumer Affairs* 45, no. 2: 248–74.

IOM (Institute of Medicine). 2007. *The Future of Drug Safety: Promoting and Protecting the Health of the Public.* Washington, DC: National Academies Press.

IOM (Institute of Medicine). 2011. *Relieving Pain in America: A Blueprint for Transforming Prevention, Care, Education, and Research.* Washington, DC: National Academies Press.

Ip, Eric J., Terrill T.-L. Tang, Vincent Cheng, and Derren S. Cheongsiatmoy. 2015. "Impact of Educational Levels and Health Literacy on Community Acetaminophen Knowledge." *Journal of Pharmacy Practice* 2, no. 6: 499–503.

Kahneman, Daniel. 2011. *Thinking, Fast and Slow.* New York: Farrar, Straus, and Giroux.

Kennedy-Hendricks, Alene, Emma E. McGinty, Colleen L. Barry. 2016. "Effects of Competing Narratives on Public Perceptions of Opioid Pain Reliever Addiction during Pregnancy." *Journal of Health Politics, Policy and Law* 41, no. 5: 873–916.

Knox, Dean, Teppei Yamamoto, Matthew A. Baum, and Adam J. Berinsky. 2019. "Design, Identification, and Sensitivity Analysis for Patient Preference Trials."

Journal of the American Statistical Association. doi.org/10.1080/01621459.2019 .1585248.

Kuehn, Bridget M. 2012. "Effects of FDA Safety Warnings May Vary." *Journal of the American Medical Association* 307, no. 9: 894–95.

Kunda, Ziva, 1990. "The Case for Motivated Reasoning." *Psychological Bulletin* 108, no. 3, 480–98.

Long, Qi, Roderick J. Little, and Xihong Lin. 2008. "Causal Inference in Hybrid Intervention Trials Involving Treatment Choice." *Journal of the American Statistical Association* 103, no. 482: 474–84.

Lupia, Arthur. 2013. "Communicating Science in Politicized Environments." *Proceedings of the National Academy of Sciences* 110, suppl. 3: 14048–54.

Mummolo, Jonathan, and Erik Peterson. 2019. "Demand Effects in Survey Experiments: An Empirical Assessment." *American Political Science Review* 113, no. 2: 517–29.

National Academies of Sciences, Engineering, and Medicine. 2017. *Pain Management and the Opioid Epidemic: Balancing Societal and Individual Benefits and Risks of Prescription Opioid Use.* Washington, DC: National Academies Press.

National Cancer Institute. 2008. "The Role of the Media in Promoting and Reducing Tobacco Use." Tobacco Control Monograph No. 19. Bethesda, MD: US Department of Health and Human Services.

Nyhan, Brendan, and Jason Reifler. 2015. "Does Correcting Myths about the Flu Vaccine Work? An Experimental Evaluation of the Effects of Corrective Information." *Vaccine* 33, no. 3: 459–64.

Orne, Martin T. 1962. "On the Social Psychology of the Psychological Experiment: With Particular Reference to Demand Characteristics and their Implications." *American Psychologist* 17, no. 11: 776–83.

Parkinson, Kristy, Joseph Price, Kosali I. Simon, and Sharon Tennyson. 2014. "The Influence of FDA Advisory Information and Black Box Warnings on Individual Use of Prescription Antidepressants." *Review of Economics of the Household* 12, no. 4: 771–90.

Regenstein, Marsha, Ellie Andres, Dylan Nelson, Stephanie David, Ruth Lopert, and Richard Katz. 2012. "Medication Information for Patients with Limited English Proficiency: Lessons from the European Union." *Journal of Law, Medicine, and Ethics* 40, no. 4: 1025–33.

Rivers, Douglas. 2006. "Understanding People: Sample Matching: Representative Sampling from Internet Panels." YouGovPolimetrix. www.websm.org/uploadi /editor/1368187057Rivers_2006_Sample_matching_Representative_sampling _from_Internet_panels.pdf (accessed January 14, 2020).

Rochella, Edward J. 2002. "The Contributions of Public Health Education toward the Reduction of Cardiovascular Disease Mortality: Experiences from the National High Blood Pressure Education Program." In *Public Health Communication,* edited by Robert C. Hornik, 73–83. Mahwah, NJ: Lawrence Erlbaum Associates.

Rücker, Gerta. 1989. "A Two-Stage Trial Design for Testing Treatment, Self-Selection, and Treatment Preference Effects." *Statistics in Medicine* 8, no. 4: 477–85. doi .wiley.com/10.1002/sim.4780080411.

Torgerson, David J., Jennifer Klaber-Moffett, and Ian T. Russell. 1996. "Patient Preferences in Randomised Trials: Threat or Opportunity?" *Journal of Health Services Research and Policy* 1, no. 4: 194–97. doi.org/10.1177/135581969600100403.

Valluri, Satish, Julie M. Zito, Daniel J. Safer, Ilene H. Zuckerman, C. Daniel Mullins, and James J. Korelitz. 2010. "Impact of the 2004 Food and Drug Administration Pediatric Suicidality Warning on Antidepressant and Psychotherapy Treatment for New-Onset Depression." *Medical Care* 48, no. 11: 947–54.

Wakefield, Melanie A., Barbara Loken, and Robert C. Hornik. 2010. "Use of Mass Media Campaigns to Change Health Behavior." *Lancet* 376, no. 9748: 1261–71.

Wolf, Michael, Jennifer King, Elizabeth A. H. Wilson, and Laura M. Curtis. 2012. "Usability of FDA-Approved Medication Guides." *Journal of General Internal Medicine* 27, no. 12: 1714–20.

Wolf, Michael S., Stacy C. Bailey, Marina Serper, Meredith Smith, Terry C. Davis, Allison L. Russell, Beenish S. Manzoor, Lisa Belter, Ruth M. Parker, and Bruce Lambert. 2014. "Comparative Effectiveness of Patient-Centered Strategies to Improve FDA Medication Guides." *Medical Care* 52, no. 9: 781–89.

Wolf, Michael S., Terry C. Davis, William H. Shrank, Marolee Neubergerd, and Ruth M. Parker. 2006. "A Critical Review of FDA-Approved Medication Guides." *Patient Education and Counseling* 62, no. 3: 316–22.

Yin, H. Shonna, Alan L. Mendelsohn, Perry Nagin, Linda van Schaick, Maria E. Cerra, and Benard P. Dreyer. 2013. "Use of Active Ingredient Information for Low Socioeconomic Status Parents' Decision-Making Regarding Cough and Cold Medications: Role of Health Literacy." *Academic Pediatrics* 13, no. 3: 229–325.

Zaller, John. 1992. *The Nature and Origins of Mass Opinion.* Cambridge: Cambridge University Press.

Why Policies Fail: The Illusion of Services in the Opioid Epidemic

Patricia Strach
University at Albany, State University of New York

Katie Zuber
John Jay College of Criminal Justice, City University of New York

Elizabeth Pérez-Chiqués
Centro de Investigación y Docencia Económicas

Abstract

Context: Although New York State is a generous provider of substance-use treatment, people who ask for help have difficulty accessing services. If the laws are on the books, the agency is there to act, and the options are available, why is treatment so hard to get?

Methods: The authors conducted 87 open-ended interviews and observed local task force meetings in Sullivan County, New York. They open coded data, identifying key topics and themes.

Findings: Even though New York is a best-case scenario for treatment, people who seek help cannot always access it. The state sees the problem as a lack of beds or information about beds, but people on the ground face real barriers that make it difficult to get treatment, including the medical model of detoxification, admissions criteria, staff shortages, and other life complications.

Conclusions: Contrary to the policy literature, this article shows that policies may fail not because they are poorly designed or implemented but because the policy itself does not address the actual underlying problem. Furthermore, in the case of opioids, it shows how misplaced solutions can hide evidence of the underlying problem, exacerbating the very issue that policy makers want to fix.

Keywords opioids, public policy, policy failure

Between 1999 and 2017, nearly 400,000 people died from opioid overdoses—roughly two-thirds of all drug-overdose deaths in the country—prompting the federal government to declare opioid use a national public health emergency (HHS 2017). In 2017, more than 3,000 New Yorkers died from an opioid overdose: a rate of 16.1 deaths per 100,000 people, which is higher than the national average of 14.6 (NIDA n.d.). Yet, New York State is a best-case scenario in terms of addressing the opioid epidemic. The state has removed major barriers to seeking treatment: It

Journal of Health Politics, Policy and Law, Vol. 45, No. 2, April 2020
DOI 10.1215/03616878-8004910   © 2020 by Duke University Press

requires licensed facilities to provide services regardless of ability to pay and forbids insurance companies from requiring preauthorization or limiting treatment to 28 days without the right to appeal. New York even has an agency dedicated specifically to substance-use services, the Office of Addiction Services and Supports (OASAS).[1] And, compared to other states, it has more public treatment options. For all of its advantages, however, we heard over and over again from people who work with or have a substance-use disorder about the difficulty accessing services. If the laws are on the books, the agency is there to act, and options are available, why is treatment so hard to get?

To answer this question, we talked to more than 80 people across New York State: policy makers in the state capital (Albany) as well as people on the frontlines of the opioid epidemic in rural Sullivan County. In discussions with local officials and families, we heard repeatedly that beds—or open slots for treatment at the doctor's office, treatment facility, or hospital—were a problem. Yet the state's online treatment locator tool showed plenty of openings, and people who worked at treatment facilities had space. We find that even in a well-resourced state like New York, services available in a database can be difficult or impossible to access in person, what we call the illusion of services. Contrary to the policy literature, we show that policies may fail not because they are poorly designed or implemented, but because the policy itself does not address the underlying problem, and, furthermore, the policy can hide evidence of the problem, exacerbating the very issue that policy makers want to fix.

Why Policies Fail: The Illusion of Services

Why do policies in place fail?[2] Existing research suggests policies fail because they may be weak, poorly designed, or poorly implemented. However, even strong, well-designed, well-implemented policies may fail if policy makers misunderstand the underlying problem.

Policies may be designed to fail. Or, at the very least, they are designed to be inefficient or ineffective to achieve other goals. Robert Saldin (2017) illustrates how—although completely unsustainable—long-term care coverage passed as part of the Affordable Care Act of 2010 not because it was sound policy (it was not), but because its inclusion *lowered* projections of the overall cost of health care. Similarly, Eva Bertram (2015) demonstrates

1. OASAS changed its name in 2019 from Office of Alcoholism and Substance Abuse Services to Office of Addiction Services and Support.
2. Our discussion here builds on the excellent work of Joseph Popcun (2018).

how expansions to the welfare state in the 1960s and 1970s came with conservative vehicles to thwart more generous policies and to permit future retrenchment. In sum, policies may be designed for purposes *other* than what their goals state.

Alternatively, policies may fail because policy makers are incentivized to please constituents rather than best address a problem. Policies with upfront preventative costs are less attractive to voters than policies that pay large amounts after the fact (Gailmard and Patty 2009), even though "investing in preparedness produces a large social benefit" (Healy and Malhotra 2009: 388). Political officials are encouraged to design poor policies because citizens and residents penalize them for taking long-term, more cost-effective action upfront.

Policies may also fail because they are poorly implemented. While top-down studies see implementation as the faithful execution of a policy's goals (Bardach 1977; Hogwood and Gunn 1997; Pressman and Wildavsky 1984; Van Meter and Van Horn 1975) and bottom-up scholars see street-level bureaucrats as policy makers, implementation scholars bridging this divide systematically lay out what may lead to better or worse imple-mentation outcomes: features of the policy, the organization and people administering it, and politics. Policy features like traceability of problems being addressed, the extent to which a statute coherently structures the implementation process, and nonstatutory variables, such as media, pub-lic support, resources, commitment, and leadership skills (Sabatier and Mazmanian 1980), are important. Administrative features matter, too, such as institutional capacity of organizations responsible for making programs work and qualifications of those people in charge (Goggin 1990) as well as conflict and ambiguity surrounding certain policy implementation deci-sions (Matland 1995). Finally, electoral, group, and administrative politics (Manna and Moffitt 2019) also play a role.

Policies may fail when the wrong solution is coupled to an existing problem. John Kingdon (1984) famously explained the three streams of the policy process: problem, politics, and policy. Policy entrepreneurs wait for a window of opportunity to open, so they may couple their desired solution to whatever problem is in the national spotlight. In the words of David Rochefort and Roger Cobb (1993: 58): "the solution begets the problem." But Kingdon, whose focus is on agenda setting, does not look at what out-comes arise when solutions do not fit the problem they are coupled with.

Researchers know that policy makers have imperfect information and foresight into what will happen in the future. Policy makers have bounded rationality, and they rely on habits and routine decision making (March and

Simon 1958; Simon 1947). Policy makers, furthermore, can be myopic, without the ability "to clearly see the horizon of the future policy environment in which impacts of the policy will develop" (Nair and Howlett 2017: 104). Given the complexity of many problems—even with the best intentions—policy makers may not affix an adequate solution to a problem. Anecdotal evidence shows misplaced policy solutions, especially in public health: cholera epidemics wrongly attributed to miasma (bad air) rather than contaminants in water (Freedman 2008) or HIV/AIDS thought to be transmitted through routine household contact rather than blood (Shilts 1987). Yet, policies may fail—even in the short term—because policy makers do not fully understand the problem and craft a solution that does not match it. As Hogwood and Gunn (1997: 219) explain, a "policy may be based upon an inadequate understanding of a problem to be solved, its causes and cure; or of an opportunity, its nature, and what is needed to exploit it" (see also Bardach 1977; Pressman and Wildavsky 1984).

In the case of New York State, we find that a well-crafted and well-implemented policy solution, the New York State OASAS bed-locator tool, does exactly what it was designed to do: keep a tally of open treatment beds in the state. But the bed-locator tool does not actually fix the problem that people on the ground face: access to these open beds. Furthermore, the tool not only gives the impression that the state has addressed the problem, it also provides data to support state officials' claims, effectively masking the real problem and thwarting efforts to address it.

A Method of Listening

Like many states, New York has an opioid problem. But, unlike many other states, New York has taken comprehensive action to address it. New York requires all state-licensed facilities to provide treatment to anyone who wants it regardless of ability to pay. The state forbids insurance pre-authorization for substance-use treatment services, and it does not allow 28-day insurance limits on treatment services without a process of appeal. Comparatively, the state has a wealth of resources, including an agency specifically devoted to substance-use services, as well as one of the largest drug-treatment systems in the United States. In 2016, New York admitted more people into state substance-use treatment programs than any other state (SAMHSA 2018). To understand why it is still difficult to access treatment, we examined rural Sullivan County, which has been heavily hit by the opioid epidemic, in greater depth.

Table 1   About Sullivan County

	Sullivan County	United States
Population	75,498	327,167,434
Non-Hispanic white	71.2%	60.4%
Household with broadband internet	76%	78.1%
High-school graduate or higher	86.4%	87.3%
Bachelor's degree or higher	23.4%	30.9%
Mean travel time to work	30.6	26.4
Median household income	$53,877	$57,652
Living in poverty	14.9%	12.3%
Land area (square miles)	968.13	3,531,905.43

Source: United States Census Bureau, www.census.gov/quickfacts/fact/table/US,sullivancounty newyork/INC110217.

Sullivan County has 75,500 residents spread across an area the size of Rhode Island. Although rural is often a mistaken euphemism for white, Sullivan has sizable African American (9.9%) and Hispanic (16.6%) populations (table 1). Roughly three-quarters of its population live in a rural part of the county, where access to health care, healthy foods, and employment is difficult. Like many rural communities across the country, Sullivan County's main industries (agriculture and tourism) receded, and the population has continued to decline.

Like many rural communities across the country, Sullivan County has a serious opioid problem. It has some of the state's highest emergency department admissions (NYSDOH 2017), highest overdose death rates (CDC Wonder n.d.), and highest opioid prescribing rates.[3] Emergency department visits and hospitalizations are higher than average for upstate New York (figure 1), and overdose deaths continue to climb (figure 2).

Why are there so many opioid-related emergency department visits? Why are deaths still on the rise? And what prevents policy makers from doing more about it?

To better understand the problem, we used a method of listening (Cramer 2016), conducting open-ended, in-depth interviews with law enforcement, lawyers, judges, providers, doctors, nurses, social workers, local government officials, activists, families, and people in recovery. Our Sullivan interviewees were identified through a stratified four-snowball sample. We started with key informants' contacts in (a) the Sullivan County Prescription

3. Prescriptions were 66.5 per 100 people in 2017, down from 106.8 in 2012. See CDC drug overdose data at www.cdc.gov/drugoverdose/maps/rxrate-maps.html.

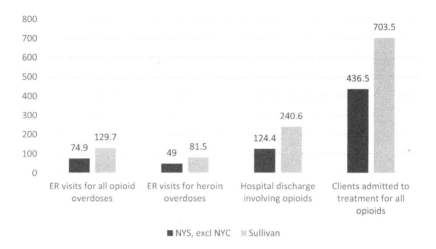

Figure 1 Sullivan opioid hospital visits per 100,000 people, 2016.

Source: Authors' analysis of the New York State Opioid Annual Data Report 2018.
Notes: Data from the New York State Department of Health (NYSDOH), www.health.ny.gov
/statistics/opioid/data/pdf/nys_opioid_annual_report_2018.pdf.

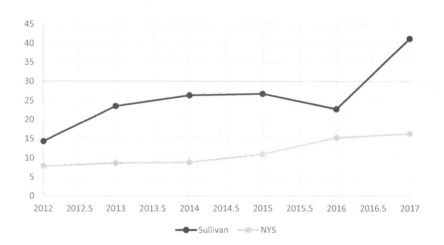

Figure 2 Overdose deaths involving any opioid per 100,000 people,
2012–17.

Source: Authors' analysis of CDC n.d.

Drug Task Force, (b) health care community, (c) activist community, and (d) local leadership. From these four starting points, we asked interviewees who else we should speak with. We also interviewed a select sample of state policy officials relevant to the opioid epidemic and elected officials representing Sullivan. Interviews lasted forty-five minutes to two hours, and most (though not all) were taped and transcribed. Between December 2017 and January 2019, for this portion of the project, we talked to 87 people in upstate New York: 46 were based in Sullivan, 20 in neighboring Orange County (where many Sullivan residents go for substance-use services), 9 in organizations that served both counties, and 12 state officials in Albany. Additionally, we attended two Sullivan County Drug Task Force meetings and two meetings of the Sullivan County Perinatal Drug Task Force, as well as public forums. We open-coded (Emerson, Fretz, and Shaw 2011) the interview data we collected, identifying key topics and themes that came up frequently in our discussions.

Our analysis revealed: (1) the appearance of services that are available on paper but unattainable in practice and (2) the disconnect between the right issue—opioid epidemic—but the wrong solutions—more beds and more information—rather than structural barriers that prevent access to treatment. In this article we discuss how one policy solution—the bed-locator tool—not only fails to help people as intended but can actually mask the underlying problem. Agency officials and providers suggest more information will help people understand the many services that are available to them. However, these additional solutions are based on an illusion of services rather than the actual problem at hand: the specific barriers that keep people from being able to access treatment when they ask for it (see, e.g., Weaver 2015).

The Beds Problem

From the first day we stepped into Sullivan County, we heard about the problem of beds in our conversations with everyone from grassroots organizers ("there are no beds" [field notes 171211]) to the Commissioner of Health and Family Services ("getting a bed is a wait" [field notes 180118]). "Beds" does not always mean physical beds. It can be, in the language of OASAS, slots in an outpatient clinic. Beds is shorthand for treatment (un)availability in the community. One local official explained, "We hear all the time they're coming and saying 'I need help,' and we are like calling everyone we could find and there's no beds anywhere to send people. . . . So, I think that to me, that there's just a lack of long-term treatment beds" (interview 42). The beds discussion also suggests the opioid problem in local communities is much bigger than the available solutions. A local health officer told us how the hospital does not have a detoxification unit, there are thirteen beds in Sullivan's main city, Monticello, a youth facility in Fallsburg, and a third facility for women. "That is it. Two others went out of business. You combine all these factors: dynamite" (interview 66).

State officials heard about a lack of beds, too. The 2016 State Heroin and Opioid Task Force, chaired by Lt. Governor Kathy Hochul and OASAS Commissioner Arlene González-Sánchez, "repeatedly heard" about a shortage of treatment beds (Heroin Opioid Task Force 2016: 13). It recommended "the State take steps to increase the number of treatment beds and expand the type of treatment beds" (Heroin Opioid Task Force 2016: 13). The governor subsequently signed into law comprehensive reforms based on the task force recommendations a mere two weeks later, including an additional 270 treatment beds and 2,335 treatment slots, adding to more than 12,500 treatment beds across New York (NYSGO 2016b). New opioid treatment programs had opened in Albany, Buffalo, the Bronx, Peekskill, Plattsburgh, Syracuse, Rome, and Watertown, while residential treatment beds were added to facilities in Staten Island, Albany, Niagara, Suffolk, and Westchester (NYSGO 2016a).

Not everybody believes that there is a bed problem. Staff at treatment facilities told us they have open beds, but people with substance-use disorders just do not know about them. At a local task force meeting we attended, the facilitator noted how difficult it is for pregnant moms to navigate the different kinds of treatment and the different rules for getting in: "There's a maze of bureaucracy. Layers upon layers of service. If the experts can't navigate it, what do you expect from these moms?" (field notes 180711). A local official also expressed frustration with how complicated it is to get help: "There's all these great programs, but what good are they if no one knows about them? . . . You can create the best program in the world, but, if no one knows about it, what good is it? There's a disconnect between the programs being offered and what people know about them" (interview 57).

OASAS, too, saw an information problem. "At OASAS we had been hearing that there were no beds available," explained an addictions specialist in an online tutorial. "So we thought there was a real need to have a quick, easy tool out there for people to be able to find beds" (OASAS 2017). The OASAS Treatment Availability Dashboard allows people to search for treatment beds across New York State based on distance, patient characteristics, and type of program. Anyone with access to the Internet can run a search, link to a description of the services offered, and download the results in a PDF file (OASAS n.d.-b). At any given time, New Yorkers can go online and see what facilities treat what kinds of addictions and whether there is space for them. "We've gotten fabulous feedback on this," explained one agency official: "I've had people email me and call me directly, telling me how wonderful it is and how it's helped them. We have many providers that are using it to find placement for clients that they can't actually serve. We've had other states contact us because they're interested in how we developed this and they'd like to create something similar in their state. So, it's been very well received" (OASAS 2017).

To further deal with what it saw as a lack of information, OASAS created an ombudsman program in 2018 to "educate individuals, families, and health care providers on their legal rights to coverage, help them to access treatment and services and . . . investigate and resolve complaints regarding denial of health insurance coverage" (OASAS 2018). In 2019, OASAS launched a "Know the Facts" campaign "to dispel myths, provide facts, and raise awareness about addiction services in New York State, and will help direct people to addiction services and help" (OASAS 2019).

For New York State's treatment providers and OASAS, both of which work day in and day out on substance use, the refrain about lack of beds is not simply an infrastructure problem, it is an information problem. Even though the bed locator can help people find treatment more easily, and even though the number of treatment beds is growing, people still struggle to get help. We asked one provider why:

> **Patricia Strach:** So, one of the things that I keep trying to figure out as I talk to folks at the state and they say "there's a thousand open beds, plus open slots, so there isn't a problem."
>
> **Nonprofit Executive:** Yeah. There's not a problem. There's open slots, yeah, there's open beds. I get emails every day from providers, "we have beds, we have beds, we have beds." Sullivan County has beds, the crisis center up there, I get emails every day from them, Catholic Charities has beds, all the providers have openings in their out-patient slots. And then we have another provider who wants to put a 200-bed rehab in the community. And I was like . . . it's not like we don't, it's like that's not the problem. That's not the problem.
>
> **Patricia Strach:** So, what is the problem? . . .
>
> **Nonprofit Executive:** I don't know, I honestly don't know. (interview 95)

How can some community members and local officials believe there are no beds available while agency officials believe there is a 1000-bed surplus? The answer is the illusion of services. Yes, there are open beds. But, no, people on the ground cannot easily access them. One mother we spoke to explained how her daughter was turned away from the same treatment facility three times—the first because her daughter was on antidepressants, the second because her daughter needed to detoxify from fentanyl, and the third time because the hospital detoxified her with methadone, which made her ineligible for a bed because the treatment facility considered methadone a drug (even though the treatment facility referred her to that hospital in a neighboring county to detoxify). Being turned away from a residential facility because of drugs may seem counterintuitive. Nonetheless, in many of these facilities patients have to be detoxed before admissions, and, in some facilities, methadone is considered a drug rather than a medication. This young woman's plight illustrates how hard it is to access services even when the bed-locator tool shows an open slot at a treatment facility.

In the next section, we lay out barriers that keep people from accessing available services—the medical model for detoxification, admissions criteria, staff shortages, and other life challenges—showing how easy it is for people who need help, like the daughter above, to be turned away. The bed-locator tool in and of itself is not a bad thing. It allows people who need services to find them. But lack of information is not the main obstacle keeping people out of treatment, lack of access is. The dashboard does not address this more difficult and intractable problem.

The Illusion of Service in the Opioid Epidemic

Why are services so hard to access? Although state officials may be right—there are plenty of treatment beds across New York—solutions like the bed-locator tool fail to address the underlying problem: concrete barriers that bar access to treatment, even when beds are available.

The Medical Model Limits Access to Hospital Services

Under federal law, hospitals are required to provide appropriate medical care for emergency medical conditions, where the absence of medical care could be expected to place the health of the individual in serious jeopardy or serious impairment to bodily functions (CMS n.d.). People who have substance-use disorders routinely go to the hospital emergency department for help. However, withdrawal is typically not treated as an emergency medical condition, and emergency care is expensive. In 2008, New York State enacted new guidelines for detoxification, shifting to a community-based model of care for withdrawal (OASAS n.d.-a). As a result, many hospitals—including Sullivan County's only hospital—do not provide detoxification services.

Most hospitals treat addiction under a medical model of care, where individuals have to be experiencing physical withdrawal before they are admitted. Essentially, people who come to the emergency department for help are sent home unless they are experiencing, as one hospital social worker described, very painful symptoms: "shakes, dilated [pupils], sweats, whole body aches, severe body aches, restlessness, it's really hard for them to stay still 'cause their aches are so bad. Body twitching, like their legs will twitch or their arms will twitch, is a sign. . . . Typically, they are nauseous, they're vomiting, they have diarrhea" (interview 65). People who have more complicated cases have a greater likelihood of being admitted to a hospital, such as patients with comorbid medical conditions, for example, diabetes or hypertension (SAMHSA 2005).

Although federal flexibility allows physicians at hospitals to treat emergency withdrawal with medications like buprenorphine, and although a state waiver allows hospitals to convert every medical bed into a detoxification bed (NYSDOH 2018), hospitals still turn patients away because they do not meet the medical criteria for withdrawal. Being admitted is so unlikely that the head of one nonprofit warns people about the difficulty. "We kind of ask [clients], because if they don't meet the admission criteria, which has nothing to do with treating addiction—it has to do with health—if they don't meet that, they are not going through an emergency room, and they're not getting into a hospital bed" (interview 95).

Prospective patients are often told to leave and come back when the symptoms are more severe. The hospital social worker above told us these conversations are difficult: "I'll say like 'come back, like, can you hang out somewhere?' [They respond:] 'I'm homeless, no car, where do you want me to go, it's winter, what am I supposed to do?' And those are valid points! Like, what are they supposed to do?" Many simply leave before they are admitted.

Admissions Criteria Limit Access to Treatment Beds

Unlike emergency departments, which are open 24 hours a day, community treatment facilities may only be open during business hours. As one provider explained, "If we have clients who work or have childcare issues, 9–5 Monday through Friday might not work" (interview 75). Yet, according to a state official, most "people don't usually say 'I want to go to treatment' Monday through Friday, 9–5" (field notes 190928). People who come for help after hours are not seen because the office is closed and there is no qualified staff member to admit them.

Even when treatment facilities are open, they do not accept every patient who comes through their doors. Facilities may turn people away if they fail to meet age or sex requirements for beds. Some beds are available only for adults whereas other beds are only available to a particular sex (male-only beds are not available to women, for example).

Treatment facilities may also turn people away if they cannot provide the appropriate level of care. For instance, not all facilities are licensed to provide medically supervised detoxification. Because withdrawal can involve complications and is often accompanied by potentially fatal side effects, treatment centers typically refer out for detoxification. But people seeking help do not always know the difference. As one local official explained, "Somebody who is experiencing addiction, or a family member who is making those calls, they can get turned away. They don't know the levels of care. It might not be the right level of care and then all of a sudden they're getting turned away because they need a higher level of care or a lower level of care, in which case they may not get into treatment" (interview 22).

People who need help may be turned away because they go to the wrong facility: they are not sick enough to be seen at an emergency department even if they are too sick or the wrong age/gender for a community treatment facility.

Staffing Shortages Make Accessing Care Difficult

Even when there are facilities with beds to treat people, severe staffing shortages mean those beds are, in practice, inaccessible to people who need them. Increased coverage for mental health means greater demand for psychologists and psychiatrists without an adequate supply (Olfson 2016). Furthermore, there are not enough physicians to provide medication-assisted treatment (MAT), which gives patients prescription drugs to block the effects of opiate withdrawal. MAT—through methadone, buprenorphine, or naltrexone—is the most effective treatment for opioid-use disorder when combined with intensive mental health and behavioral counseling.

Yet, more than half of US counties lack physicians who can prescribe buprenorphine, leaving 30 million people without access (Rosenblatt et al. 2015).

The staff problem is widespread: a lack of social workers, credentialed alcoholism and substance abuse counselors (CASACs), and nurse practitioners. Half of agencies specializing in substance use say they have difficulty filling open positions, primarily because of a lack of qualified applicants (Hoge et al. 2013, citing Ryan, Murphy, and Krom 2012). Turnover is high (19% nationally, but 40% in some reports) because of low pay, few benefits, and heavy caseloads, as well as the stigma of working with addictions (Hoge et al. 2013). In Sullivan, social workers can carry caseloads of 70 or 80 clients (interview 60).

Staff shortages mean that beds can remain empty. A nonprofit worker in neighboring Orange County, whose job it is to connect clients to services, explained how one local treatment facility "is a great place. Clients are really happy with the treatment." But, as much as she would like to place people there, "no one is answering the phone. You have to leave a message, and nobody gets back to you" (field notes 180711). If there is no receptionist to answer the phone or nurse to do intake, people who need help cannot get it at the facility regardless of what the bed-locator tool indicates.

The problem is not lack of beds, but staff shortages that make those beds unavailable to people who ask for help. As one person who worked for a nonprofit provider explained, "This is the frustration of the treatment programs . . . they keep expanding access to treatment, but you can't find a nurse practitioner to write buprenorphine" (interview 51). What few people there are who specialize in addiction services are hard to hire, and county governments and nonprofits cannot compete with hospitals and for-profit providers who can afford to pay higher salaries. Unable to offer a competitive salary, Sullivan County had difficulty filling five vacancies including four social work positions and a CASAC position. The county cannot pay well, because, as one government official observed, you "can't get something out of a dry well" (interview 60).

Although federal rules and regulations could alleviate the problem of staff shortages—by incentivizing people to pursue training as addiction specialists, for example—existing policies do just the opposite: they make it harder for people to find a provider who can prescribe MAT. Under existing law, physicians, dentists, veterinarians, physician assistants, nurse practitioners, and nurse midwives in New York can prescribe opioids, but MAT requires specialized clinics, trainings, and authorization. Methadone is a Schedule II drug, available only through highly regulated clinics, which patients have to visit daily when they first start methadone maintenance. Buprenorphine, a Schedule III drug, can be prescribed in physicians' offices, but it requires practitioners to obtain a DEA waiver, which includes an 8-hour training for doctors and an additional 16 hours of online training for physicians' assistants and nurse practitioners (CRS 2019). Ironically, it is far easier to prescribe opioids than the medication-assisted treatment to help people stop using them. As one state official explained, "If you want pills, limp into the ER and when they ask you how much pain you have say seven and you'll get it. But if you want methadone it's regulated as if it were weapons-grade plutonium. Clinics have to keep it in a huge safe. A vault. It prevents access" (field notes 190928).

In addition to limiting which medical personnel can provide MAT, federal regulations also limit how many patients they can treat. During the first year of buprenorphine certification, physicians can have up to 30 patients under treatment at one time. After a year, they can apply to have the number increased to 100, then 275 (SAMHSA n.d.-b). In 2016, less than 4% of physicians were waivered to prescribe buprenorphine in the US (Wakeman and Rich 2018). Of the 55,000 physicians who can prescribe buprenorphine in the US, 72% are 30-Patient Certified, 20% are 100-Patient Certified, and 8% are 275-Patient Certified (SAMHSA n.d.-c). Even if every physician prescribed at the limit there would still be more patients than treatment slots. But most physicians do not prescribe to the limit (Jones, Campopiano, and McCance-Katz 2015). More than 30 million people (10% of the population) do not have access to a single prescriber of medications for addiction treatment—the overwhelming majority (21 million) are in rural areas (Rosenblatt et al. 2015).

Other Life Challenges Make Accessing Treatment Difficult

Other life and logistical challenges make it hard to access treatment, too. Family obligations can be an impediment to care. Mothers are particularly hard to get into inpatient treatment because they do not want to leave their children. As one local official explained,

> It's easier to take a male out of a home than a female, especially as far as caregivers. When we try to treat women[, it] is very difficult for us to get them to comply with any level, or any higher level of care anywhere, 'cause they don't want to leave their kids and their responsibilities

and everything they have to do. Not saying that men don't feel the same way. But, for some reason, we can leverage them a little bit easier (interview 60).

Sullivan County is fortunate to have a women-only facility, which takes pregnant women and women with children younger than 3 years old. Many mothers, however, have children older than that.

Lack of transportation, too, makes it difficult for people who suffer from addiction to get the services they need. Transportation came up in 32 of our interviews. Medicaid will pay for taxis to medical appointments but not to the pharmacy, grocery store, or work. One person explained, "Access to just normal health care is really limited and . . . that's even aggravated substantially by the distances that people need to travel. So, you may live in like Cochecton or wherever and it's 40 minutes to Monticello, and there's probably no primary care physician closer, you know, so that creates an issue for people" (interview 32).

Mental health issues are also a barrier to access. Even though substance use frequently co-occurs with mental health disorders—in 2017, 18.7 million American adults had a substance-use disorder, and 45.6% of them (8.5 million people) also had a co-occurring mental illness (SAMHSA n.d.-a)—mental health providers will often reject someone with a substance-use disorder, and substance-use providers will often reject someone with a mental health issue because of the complications medications like benzodiazepines and opioids present (interview 49). One doctor described it this way: "It's like a house with two fires. Fire is the addiction. The second is the psychiatric co-morbidity. You have to put out both fires for this to work" (field notes 190927). Yet, it rarely works. Only half of people who have a substance-use disorder or mental health issue receive treatment for either, but a small fraction receive treatment for both (HHS 2018).

Although New York State eliminated some of the most daunting limitations on access—such as ability to pay and some insurance restrictions—even in this well-resourced state, we have found an illusion of services: beds are available in the OASAS system, but people on the ground cannot access them. The illusion can be difficult to combat because computer systems show capacity to treat patients even when capacity is not there (lack of staff, limits on how many people health care professionals can and will treat). Furthermore, patients may be turned away because they do not meet the demographic characteristics, they have co-occurring conditions, or they simply choose to forgo treatment because they are stymied by family or transportation issues.

When Policies Are Created Based on a Disconnect

New York State lawmakers have not shied away from addressing the opioid epidemic. In 2012, New York created a prescription monitoring program (I-STOP), requiring real-time data reporting ("Duty to Consult," Chapter 447 of NYS Laws 2012; Heroin and Opioid Task Force 2016). In 2014, the state passed comprehensive legislation to address opioids, including initiatives for new state police officers, increased criminal penalties for selling narcotics, insurance regulations to make care easier to access, and a public education campaign (NYSGO 2014). It passed comprehensive legislation, based on the Heroin and Opioid Task Force recommendations, again in 2016.

Still, addressing beds has been a large part of the state's strategy. The state's two-pronged approach of expanding the total number of treatment beds and creating a bed locator may have enhanced treatment supply and provided information to the community, but it does not necessarily address the fundamental reasons people do not get treatment. As we have shown, people face very specific barriers: a medical model of detoxification, admissions criteria, staff shortages, and life challenges. In other words, the gulf between what officials believe to be the problem (lack of beds or information about beds) and what actually causes it (structural barriers) undermines the effectiveness of their solutions. So why have state policy makers and officials focused on beds and information instead?

There are many potential reasons why legislators and executive agency officials might address the problem as we have explained it here. First and foremost, treatment is expensive, and people who are dependent on drugs are not a well-regarded target population (Schneider and Ingram 1993). Lack of action may reflect lack of interest. Interest, however, does not seem to be a problem in New York. Although the state could certainly do more to address opioids in local communities, it provided treatment services to approximately 234,000 individuals in 2015 (OASAS 2016) and, in 2016, allocated (from all government sources, including Medicaid) over $1.4 billion for OASAS to address the crisis (Heroin Opioid Task Force 2016: 2).

Alternatively, organizational logic could have driven behavior in one of two ways. Agency officials at OASAS may have simplified the problem so that it could be addressed with an administratively easy and inexpensive solution (Scott 1998), or policy makers could have used standard modes of addressing problems, based as much on habits and routines as specific analysis of a particular problem (March and Simon 1958; Simon 1947). But here, too, it seems unlikely because New York has taken a broad range of actions: legislative solutions with comprehensive reforms in 2014 and 2016 and executive agencies expanding Medicaid under the 2010 Affordable Care Act to ensure that every New Yorker can afford drug treatment.

Finally, legislators may have misunderstood what constituencies across the state want and, in return, what the appropriate state reaction might be (Brookman and Skovron 2018; Hertel-Fernandez, Mildenberger, and Stokes 2018), either because they chose to listen to interest groups over citizens (Gilens and Page 2014), or because some communities were better able to convey their concerns as more important over others (Konisky and Reenock 2013). In our discussions with local officials, providers, and community members in Sullivan, we heard repeated, unprompted references to a disconnect between what communities say is the problem and what policy makers hear. One local official explained, "There's a disconnect between what the community provides and what the state believes." The official continued,

> So now you have the state talking to the county. But yet, the information that's down here, the people that are in the trenches, doesn't get up there. It just doesn't. And then they make decisions based on a disconnect. And then people scream loud enough and in 10–20 years we come back around and are having the same argument all over again. . . . I really think they need to turn off their brains, turn on their ears. (interview 60)

Although political scientists have shown that elected officials misperceive public opinion (Brookman and Skovron 2018; Hertel-Fernandez, Mildenberger, and Stokes 2018), the disconnect this official describes may reflect a broader lack of understanding about the concrete challenges people seeking treatment face and a broader inability to address the real problem. Even though state policy makers have not shied away from the epidemic, people on the frontlines feel as though the "money's being wasted" (interview 14).

Conclusion

Policies fail for many reasons, including poor design and/or poor implementation. In this article, we show that even a well-designed and well-implemented policy can fail when it does not address the underlying problem. We documented how beds, which are supposedly open per the computer screen, are not accessible to people who show up at the door, what we call the illusion of services. Although the state has put resources into creating beds and a bed-locator tool to provide information, these solutions do not address some of the main reasons why individuals who want help cannot get it: concrete barriers that limit access. In the case of the opioid epidemic in New York, the bed-locator tool provides data about a surplus of available help, but that help is unavailable to people who try to access it.

Although the bed-locator tool can be a valuable part of a broader strategy, it can also mask the true problem. It creates an illusion of services. Agency officials can point to open beds, and they believe that help is available when it is not. For example, in a conversation with an agency official we gave examples of what we have heard on the frontlines, including the following:

> **Patricia Strach:** We talked to a mom, she's been in this 15 years, and we said, "Well, you know, what supports are there?" And she walked out of the room and then came back after she composed herself and said, "There's nothing."
> **OASAS Official:** There is.

The illusion of services can be more frustrating than having no services at all. In the case of the latter, it is clear what is not available and what people do not have access to. But it is exasperating to people on the frontlines of the opioid epidemic to see services that are supposedly available be just out of reach. The experience can fuel the idea of a disconnect between the governmental response and what people in communities need. As one mother put it, "Stop putting information out there where it looks like you're doing something and you're really not. . . . Stop the bullshit" (interview 14).

The illusion of services can prevent policy makers from putting the right solutions in place. To end the illusion, policy makers could target solutions to address specific problems that prevent more people from getting the help they need. First, policy makers could address the medical model of care by ensuring each county has a detoxification facility with easy and open access. Facilities might be the local hospital emergency department, which would be required to take patients needing detoxification services, or they could be a dedicated 24-7 building. Policy makers could create and enforce standard protocols for treating substance-use disorder in medical facilities, much like standard protocols for chest pain. Second, policy makers could address admissions criteria that lead community facilities to turn patients away, creating a *system* of care so everyone who asks for help is able to receive it. Third, policy makers could address staffing needs by incentivizing people to go into addiction-related specializations, especially in underserved areas (including rural communities). State policy makers could work with federal policy makers to standardize regulations on opioids and MAT, so it would not be easier to prescribe opioids than the medication to help people with opioid-use disorder. Fourth, state policy makers could reduce the barriers that people with co-occurring conditions face (hospitals should be able to treat these). Solutions like these, however, will be hard to pursue as long as the illusion of services is in place.

In this article, we examined substance-use treatment in Sullivan County. Yet, the concept of illusion of services is applicable to a broad array of failures in public-service provision, especially fragmented policy areas like health. For example, a guarantee for reproductive health services means very little if there are few or no clinics in a state or doctors to perform procedures (Dresser 2008; Feleder et al. 2019). Furthermore, the disconnect people feel between what government provides and what they need is not limited to Sullivan. In our broader research, we heard about a disconnect from people on the frontlines of the opioid epidemic in New York City, Syracuse, and Albany, too.

Not being able to access services is a problem. But with opioids, the consequences are especially dire. Every time someone is turned away from a supposedly available bed, the community loses an opportunity to save a life. The illusion of services means that people who try—and fail—to access services are invisible to state officials making public policies. The state-run systems to track treatment services show open slots, whether or not people on the ground can actually access them. Policies may be well designed and executed but they do not address—and in some cases exacerbate—a broader problem that policy makers wish to fix.

■ ■ ■

Patricia Strach is a professor in the Departments of Political Science and Public Administration and Policy at the University at Albany, State University of New York, and is the interim executive director of the Rockefeller Institute of Government. pstrach@albany.edu

Katie Zuber is a doctoral lecturer in political science at John Jay College of Criminal Justice and a fellow at the Rockefeller Institute of Government.

Elizabeth Pérez Chiqués is an assistant professor at Centro de Investigación y Docencia Económicas (CIDE) and a fellow at the Rockefeller Institute of Government. Her research interests center on corruption and public personnel management.

Acknowledgments

We thank the people on the frontlines in Sullivan and Orange Counties and the state officials in Albany for giving their time and for sharing their stories with us. We also thank the attendees at the Politics of the Opioid Epidemic conference, the Politics and History Group at the University at Albany, the *JHPPL* reviewers for their helpful comments, and the Rockefeller Institute of Government for supporting this project. Any errors are our own.

References

Bardach, Eugene. 1977. *The Implementation Game: What Happens after a Bill Becomes a Law.* Cambridge, MA: MIT Press.

Bertram, Eva. 2015. *The Workfare State: Public Assistance Politics from the New Deal to the New Democrats.* Philadelphia: University of Pennsylvania Press.

Brookman, David E., and Christopher Skovron. 2018. "Bias in Perceptions of Public Opinion among Political Elites." *American Political Science Review* 112, no. 3: 542–63.

CDC (Centers for Disease Control and Prevention). n.d. "Multiple Cause of Death Data." CDC Wonder. wonder.cdc.gov/mcd.html (accessed November 13, 2019).

CMS (Centers for Medicare and Medicaid Services). 2012. "Emergency Medical Treatment and Labor Act (EMTALA)." March 26. www.cms.gov/Regulations-and -Guidance/Legislation/EMTALA/index.html.

Cramer, Katherine J. 2016. *The Politics of Resentment: Rural Consciousness in Wisconsin and the Rise of Scott Walker.* Chicago: University of Chicago Press.

CRS (Congressional Research Service). 2019. "Opioid Treatment Programs and Related Federal Regulations." June 12. fas.org/sgp/crs/misc/IF10219.pdf.

Dresser, Rebecca. 2008. "From Double Standard to Double Bind: Informed Choice in Abortion Law." *George Washington Law Review* 76, no. 6: 1599–622. www.gwlr .org/wp-content/uploads/2012/08/76-6-Dresser.pdf.

Emerson, Robert M., Rachel I. Fretz, and Linda L. Shaw. 2011. *Writing Ethnographic Fieldnotes.* 2nd ed. Chicago: University of Chicago Press.

Feleder, Florencia, Katie Gowing, Kadie Mendez, Vanessa Taylor, and Megan Weiss. 2019. "Beyond Roe: The State of Sexual and Reproductive Healthcare in New York State." Rockefeller Institute of Government, January 2. rockinst.org/issue-area /beyond-roe-the-state-of-sexual-and-reproductive-healthcare-in-new-york-state.

Freedman, David A. 2008. "On Types of Scientific Enquiry: The Role of Qualitative Reasoning." In *The Oxford Handbook of Political Methodology*, edited by Janet M. Box-Steffensmeier, Henry E. Brady, and David Collier, 300–18. New York: Oxford University Press.

Gailmard, Sean W., and John W. Patty. 2018. "Preventing Prevention." *American Journal of Political Science* 63, no. 2: 342–52. doi.org/10.1111/ajps.12411.

Gilens, Martin, and Benjamin I. Page. 2014. "Testing Theories of American Politics: Elites, Interest Groups, and Average Citizens." *Perspectives on Politics* 12, no. 3: 564–81.

Goggin, Malcolm L. 1990. *Implementation Theory and Practice: Toward a Third Generation.* Glenville, IL: Scott Foresman and Co.

Healy, Andrew, and Neil Malhotra. 2009. "Myopic Voters and Natural Disaster Policy." *American Political Science Review* 103, no. 3: 387–406.

Heroin and Opioid Task Force, State of New York. 2016. "Combatting the Heroin and Opioid Crisis: Heroin and Opioid Task Force Report." June 9. www.governor.ny .gov/sites/governor.ny.gov/files/atoms/files/HeroinTaskForceReport_3.pdf.

Hertel-Fernandez, Alexander, Matto Mildenberger, and Leah C. Stokes. 2018. "Legislative Staff and Representation in Congress." *American Political Science Review* 113, no. 1: 1–18.

HHS (US Department of Health and Human Services). 2017. "HHS Acting Secretary Declares Public Health Emergency to Address National Opioid Crisis." October 26. www.hhs.gov/about/news/2017/10/26/hhs-acting-secretary-declares-public-health -emergency-address-national-opioid-crisis.html.

HHS (US Department of Health and Human Services), Office of the Surgeon General. 2018. *Facing Addiction in America: The Surgeon General's Spotlight on Opioids.* Washington, DC: US Department of Health and Human Services.

Hoge, Michael A., Gail W. Stuart, John Morris, Michael T. Flaherty, Manuel Paris Jr., and Eric Goplerud. 2013. "Mental Health and Addiction Workforce Development: Federal Leadership Is Needed to Address the Growing Crisis." *Health Affairs* 32, no. 11: 2005–12.

Hogwood, Brian, and Lewis Gunn. 1997. "Why 'Perfect Implementation' is Unattainable." In *The Policy Process: A Reader*, edited by Michael Hill, 217–25. New York: Routledge.

Jones, Christopher M., Melinda Campopiano, Grant Baldwin, and Elinore McCance-Katz. 2015. "National and State Treatment Need and Capacity for Opioid Agonist Medication-Assisted Treatment." *American Journal of Public Health* 105, no. 8: e55–e63.

Kingdon, John. 1984. *Agendas, Alternatives, and Public Policies.* Boston: Little, Brown, and Company.

Konisky, David, and Christopher Reenock. 2013. "Examining Sources of Compliance Bias in Policy Implementation." *Journal of Politics* 75, no. 2: 506–19.

March, James G., and Herbert Simon. 1958. *Organizations.* New York: Free Press.

Manna, Paul, and Susan L. Moffitt. 2019. "Traceable Tasks and Complex Policies: When Politics Matter for Policy Implementation." *Policy Studies Journal*, June 17. doi.org/10.1111/psj.12348.

Matland, Richard E. 1995. "Synthesizing the Implementation Literature: The Ambiguity-Conflict Model of Policy Implementation." *Journal of Public Administration Research and Theory* 5, no. 2: 145–74.

Nair, Sreeja, and Michael Howlett. 2017. "Policy Myopia as a Source of Policy Failure: Adaptation and Policy Learning under Deep Uncertainty." *Policy and Politics* 45, no. 1: 103–18.

NIDA (National Institute on Drug Abuse). 2019. "Opioid-Involved Overdose Deaths."
New York Opioid Summary, March. www.drugabuse.gov/opioid-summaries-by
-state/new-york-opioid-summary.

NYSDOH (New York State Department of Health). 2017. *Opioid Annual Report*.
October. www.health.ny.gov/statistics/opioid/data/pdf/nys_opioid_annual_report_
2017.pdf.

NYSDOH (New York State Department of Health). 2018. DAL 18-05: "Time Limited
Waiver to Provide Detoxification Services in Excess of Bed/Patient Days Thresh-
olds." March 2. www.health.ny.gov/professionals/hospital_administrator/letters
/2018/2018-03-02_dhdtc_dal_18-05_waiver_detox_services.htm.

NYSGO (New York State Governor's Office). 2014. "Governor Cuomo Signs Legislation to Combat Heroin, Opioid, and Prescription Drug Abuse Epidemic." June
24. www.governor.ny.gov/news/governor-cuomo-signs-legislation-combat-heroin
-opioid-and-prescription-drug-abuse-epidemic-0.

NYSGO (New York State Governor's Office). 2016a. "Governor Cuomo Announces
Expanded Online Tool to Connect New Yorkers to Addiction Treatment Services."
December 6. www.governor.ny.gov/news/governor-cuomo-announces-expanded
-online-tool-connect-new-yorkers-addiction-treatment-services.

NYSGO (New York State Governor's Office). 2016b. "Governor Cuomo Signs Legislation to Combat the Heroin and Opioid Crisis." June 22. www.governor.ny.gov
/news/governor-cuomo-signs-legislation-combat-heroin-and-opioid-crisis.

OASAS (New York State Office of Alcoholism and Substance Abuse Services). n.d.-a.
"Medically Managed Detoxification Reform." www.oasas.ny.gov/admin/hcf
/mmdreform.cfm (accessed October 24, 2019).

OASAS (New York State Office for Alcoholism and Substance Abuse Services). n.d.-b.
"Treatment Availability Dashboard." findaddictiontreatment.ny.gov/ (accessed
October 24, 2019).

OASAS (New York State Office of Alcoholism and Substance Abuse Services). 2016.
Statewide Comprehensive Report 2015–2019. www.oasas.ny.gov/pio/commissioner
/documents/OASASStatewidePlan20152019.pdf (accessed October 24, 2019).

OASAS (New York State Office of Alcoholism and Substance Abuse Services). 2017.
"Learn about the Treatment Availability Dashboard." May 11. www.youtube.com
/watch?v=mkdfnQFhEmA.

OASAS (New York State Office of Alcoholism and Substance Abuse Services).
2018. "OMH, OASAS, and DFS Announce New Program and Regulations to Help
New Yorkers Access Insurance Coverage for Substance Abuse and Mental Health
Services." October 19. apps.cio.ny.gov/apps/mediaContact/public/view.cfm?parm=
7B67BF05–0A7F-7047–33DF96DD8A99F9CE&backButton.

OASAS (New York State Office of Alcoholism and Substance Abuse Services). 2019.
"New York State Office of Alcoholism and Substance Abuse Services Announces
New Campaign." February 11. www.oasas.ny.gov/pio/press/20190211OASAS
Announcesknowthefactscampaign.cfm.

Olfson, Mark. 2016. "Building the Mental Health Workforce Capacity Needed to Treat
Adults with Serious Mental Illnesses." *Health Affairs* 35, no. 6: 983–90. doi.org/
10.1377/hlthaff.2015.1619.

Popcun, Joseph. 2018. "Defining and Understanding Ordinary Failures in Public Policy." Unpublished paper.

Pressman, Jeffrey, and Aaron Wildavsky. 1984. *Implementation: How Great Expectations in Washington Are Dashed in Oakland*. Berkeley: University of California Press.

Rochefort, David A., and Roger W. Cobb. 1993. "Problem Definition, Agenda Access, and Policy Choice." *Policy Studies Journal* 21, no. 1: 56–71.

Rosenblatt, Roger A., C. Holly A. Andrilla, Mary Catlin, and Eric H. Larson. 2015. "Geographic and Specialty Distribution of US Physicians Trained to Treat Opioid Use Disorder." *Annals of Family Medicine* 13, no. 1: 23–26.

Ryan, Olivia, Deena Murphy, and Laurie Krom. 2012. *Vital Signs: Taking the Pulse of the Addiction Treatment Workforce, A National Report, Version 1*. Kansas City, MO: Addiction Technology Transfer Center National Office in residence at the University of Missouri-Kansas City.

Sabatier, Paul, and Daniel Mazmanian. 1980. "The Implementation of Public Policy: A Framework of Analysis." *Policy Studies Journal* 8, no. 4: 538–60.

Saldin, Robert P. 2017. *When Bad Policy Makes Good Politics*. New York: Oxford University Press.

SAMHSA (Substance Abuse and Mental Health Services Administration). n.d.-a. "Key Substance Use and Mental Health Indicators in the United States: Results from the 2017 National Survey on Drug Use and Health." September. www.samhsa.gov/data/sites/default/files/cbhsq-reports/NSDUHFFR2017/NSDUHFFR2017.pdf (accessed November 13, 2019).

SAMHSA (Substance Abuse and Mental Health Services Administration). n.d.-b. "Apply for a Practitioner Waiver." www.samhsa.gov/medication-assisted-treatment/buprenorphine-waiver-management/increase-patient-limits (accessed October 24, 2019).

SAMHSA (Substance Abuse and Mental Health Services Administration). n.d.-c. "Practitioner and Program Data." www.samhsa.gov/programs-campaigns/medication-assisted-treatment/training-materials-resources/physician-program-data (accessed October 24, 2019).

SAMHSA (Substance Abuse and Mental Health Services Administration). 2005. "Substance Abuse Treatment for Persons With Co-Occurring Disorders." Treatment Improvement Protocol (TIP) Series 42, Report No. (SMA) 05-3992. www.ncbi.nlm.nih.gov/books/NBK64197/ (accessed October 24, 2019).

SAMHSA (Substance Abuse and Mental Health Services Administration). 2018. "Treatment Episode Data Set (TEDS) 2016: Admissions to and Discharges from Publicly Funded Substance Use Treatment." August. www.samhsa.gov/data/sites/default/files/2016_Treatment_Episode_Data_Set_Annual.pdf.

Schneider, Anne, and Helen Ingram. 1993. "Social Construction of Target Populations: Implications for Politics and Policy." *American Political Science Review* 87, no. 2: 334–37.

Scott, James. 1998. *Seeing Like a State: How Certain Schemes to Improve the Human Condition Have Failed*. New Haven, CT: Yale University Press.

Shilts, Randy. 1987. *And The Band Played on: Politics, People, and the AIDS Epidemic.* New York: St. Martin's Press.

Simon, Herbert A. 1947. *Administrative Behavior.* New York: MacMillan.

Van Meter, Donald, and Carl Van Horn. 1975. "The Policy Implementation Process: A Conceptual Framework." *Administration and Society* 6, no. 4: 445–88.

Wakeman, Sarah E., and Josiah D. Rich. 2018. "Barriers to Medications for Addiction Treatment: How Stigma Kills." *Substance Use and Misuse* 53, no. 2: 330–33. doi.org/10.1080/10826084.2017.1363238.

Weaver, R. Kent. 2015. "Getting People to Behave: Research Lessons for Policy Makers." *Public Administration Review* 75, no. 6: 806–16.

Commentary

Framing, Governance, and Partisanship: Putting Politics Front and Center in the Opioid Epidemic

Miriam J. Laugesen
Columbia University

Eric M. Patashnik
Brown University

The opioid epidemic ranks as one of the most serious and tragic public health crises in US history. The cost in human lives, health care, and lost work productivity is staggering. While there are signs that the opioid epidemic may have begun to level off, tens of thousands of opioid deaths continue to occur every year.

The roots of the United States' opioid epidemic are generally well known. Beginning in the 1990s, physicians, pressured by aggressive and deceptive marketing by pharmaceutical companies, began prescribing opioids widely to reduce the suffering of acute and chronic pain, which had long been seen as neglected. Misuse of opioids and drug addiction (despite promises from drug companies that the risk of abuse was low) increased dramatically. In subsequent waves of the crisis, many opioid users began turning to illicit opioids including heroin and synthetic drugs like fentanyl. The crisis has devastated communities and millions of families across the United States. Many academic studies and government commission reports have focused on education, treatment, and other strategies to address the opioid epidemic. Progress is being made, but the crisis will continue for many years to come.

While the actions of pharmaceutical companies, drug distributors, and "pill mill" physicians are the proximate cause of the opioid epidemic, public policy is also implicated in the crisis. Government is charged with regulating the marketing of prescription drugs, enforcing laws against the consumption and sale of illegal drugs, and promoting public health. The failure of policy makers to recognize the severity of the crisis as it was

Journal of Health Politics, Policy and Law, Vol. 45, No. 2, April 2020
DOI 10.1215/03616878-8004958   © 2020 by Duke University Press

emerging and to act in a timely and appropriate manner by providing treatment services to at-risk populations and other necessary interventions must be considered in any effort to understand the scale of the epidemic's toll. The articles in this special issue fill that gap, and offer a broader perspective on the role of health politics and policy in the opioid crisis. The contributors explore the political, cultural, and institutional context in which the epidemic grew into the nation's most serious public health threat and in which ongoing responses are being designed and implemented. The issue offers many lessons for scholars interested in the intersection of population health, law, politics, and governance.

One of the most striking characteristics of these essays is the multidimensional nature of the issue. There is no single opioid crisis but rather multiple distinct causes as well as many different problematizations and interpretations of the impact of the introduction of these new compounds into the health care system. The contributors explore the role of different actors, including the public, the states, the media, Congress, and the bureaucracy (as well as their interactions) to understand how good intentions to reduce pain-related suffering, financial incentives, and policy breakdowns coincide. Three core themes emerge from the essays. The first is the powerful role of narratives and framing in shaping understandings of the opioid epidemic. The second is the opioid epidemic as a test of healthcare system governance. The third theme is the role of partisanship in mediating responses to the crisis.

The Role of Framing in the Opioid Epidemic

There is no one correct or natural way to understand the opioid epidemic. How people understand it—and how they apprise the benefits and costs of different ways to address it—are shaped by the political context in which discussions about the epidemic take place. It is clear that in such discussions words matter, and that it is impossible to even conceive of the politics or policy response without considering the narrative and framing, or how we describe it (pain management, drug abuse, public health epidemic). At the same time, unlike some policy phenomena, there is the undisputed fact of large-scale mortality and morbidity. The opioid epidemic for many years was *under-* rather than overstated, and the opposite of what Goode and Ben-Yehuda (1994) describe as a moral panic. Given that, it seems justifiable to agree with the nature of this as a bona fide crisis.

Several of the essays in this issue build on the rich traditions from different fields regarding the influence of framing on how we think about problems (leading scholars in this tradition include Peter L. Berger and

Thomas Luckmann [1966], Anne Schneider and Helen Ingram [1993], and Deborah Stone [2011], to name just a few). That intellectual tradition demands that the opioid crisis be seen as a policy or political phenomenon with a social construction. Only by disaggregating the phenomenon, and by recognizing the hidden assumptions that anchor its conceptualization, can we truly understand how a problem even comes to be seen as such.

In their essay comparing media representations of the crack cocaine and opioid epidemics, Carmel Shachar, Tess Wise, Gail Katznelson, and Andrea Louise Campbell point out that "the model used to frame a substance abuse epidemic is crucial because it not only shapes public perception of the epidemic but also the public policy responses." The authors show that newspaper articles on the opioid epidemic are more likely to use medical terminology (such as health, treatment, and overdose) and that articles on the crack cocaine epidemic are more likely to use the language of social control and criminal justice (such as police, enforcement, and arrest). The differential framing of the two epidemics shows that race may play a contributing role in media framing. This is consistent with past research recognizing how some issues, such as welfare, have been racialized and closely identified with African American populations (Gilens 1999). However, the authors' finding that coverage of the methamphetamine epidemic also involved a criminal justice narrative suggests that the different framing of opioids and crack cocaine does not merely result from the different racial group predominately affected. The authors further show that while coverage of heroin shifted toward a medical frame over time, the tone and content of coverage of heroin still differed from coverage of opioids. This disparity suggests that another dimension that affects the framing of coverage is whether or not the drug in question is illegal. The authors make a strong case that in order for a media narrative to shift, two factors must come together: "an overall reframing of substance use as a public health issue" and "a perception that most users of the particular substance are white." Taken together, the findings of the article offer new insights into how racial factors interact with other elements of the political and policy context to shape issue framing.

The essay by Jin Woo Kim, Evan Morgan, and Brendan Nyhan provides further evidence that perceptions of the racial identity of victims mediates political responses to public health epidemics. Examining sponsorship of drug-related bills in the US House of Representatives and drug-related mortality data at the district level, the authors find that legislators were more likely to introduce punitive legislation during the crack epidemic, whereas they are more likely to introduce treatment-oriented legislation during the opioid epidemic. Further, the authors show that legislators respond to drug deaths in their districts by sponsoring more treatment-oriented legislation, but "this relationship is only observed for opioid deaths and white victims." Once again, we see how words are not just about words; framing likely reflects—and amplifies—preexisting racial inequity in society.

The essays in this issue not only explore how race mediates policy responses but also shed light on how issues like the opioid crisis come to be racialized in the first place, particularly when the victims are predominately white. Although the opioid epidemic is commonly described by public health experts as a major cause of the white "deaths of despair" hypothesis (Case and Deaton 2015), it is not obvious that opioids would necessarily be seen as a white issue—perhaps like the tendency of whites to not describe themselves in racial terms, thinking as they do, as the default rather than the exception in categories. Conversely, "people of color are almost always seen as 'having a race' . . . whereas whites are rarely defined by race" (DiAngelo 2012: 175). Indeed, the lack of initial racialization of the crisis raises questions that scholars may debate for a number of years into the future, but, at least for now, scholars in this issue provide some guideposts for exploration.

In their essay, Sarah E. Gollust and Joanne M. Miller examine whether the perception that whites are faring comparatively poorly in the opioid epidemic shapes white views on how to address it. Using a survey experiment, the authors show that white subjects who saw a news article framed to emphasize the higher rate of opioid mortality among whites increased whites' perception that they are on the losing side in the health policy domain. This loser perception, in turn, makes whites less supportive of government policies that are empathetic to opioid users, such as prevention programs and efforts to reduce stigma. In short, social identity is a key mediator of public opinion, and whites' willingness to support policies that would arguably help their own health and well-being depends on how whites view their position in society relative to nonwhites. These findings should encourage further scholarship into the ways (both intended and unintended) that elite messaging can create a perception that one group is winning and another is losing, even when public health policies would benefit the population as a whole.

The Opioid Epidemic and Healthcare Governance

Both policy makers and scholars may describe phenomena such as the opioid crisis as an aberration, as an unforeseen and novel governance challenge, perhaps as a way to explain flat-footed responses. In fact, crises such as the opioid crisis are a test of the resilience or "stress tests" for governance. Natural disasters like hurricanes and earthquakes are such tests. They reveal the adequacy of infrastructure investment and the quality and level of compliance with building codes, for example. Similarly, a health care system must have the capacity to meet new epidemics and other challenges, sometimes much more quickly than expected.

The scale of the opioid crisis in the United States—the fact that so many people have been caught in its grip for so many years—is taken by some as prima facie evidence of indicator of poor performance of American government. Yet many questions remain about just *why* government's response to the opioid epidemic has been so sluggish and inadequate. Governance failures can arise from multiple and reinforcing causes, including institutional fragmentation that prevents policy coordination, inadequate spending on vital public services, special-interest influence that diverts policy goals away from the common good, the short time horizons of reelection-minded officials, and implementation breakdowns of various kinds.

No doubt these and other factors have been at play in the opioid case. As Patricia Strach, Katie Zuber, and Elizabeth Peréz-Chiqués show in their article on treatment policies in New York State, however, government's actions can make a public health crisis worse, even when policies are well crafted and do what they are intended to do, because they are based on a faulty definition of the underlying problem. The authors' decision to study New York State is interesting because it offers a best-case scenario—a jurisdiction with the political will to address the opioid crisis and a higher level of institutional and administrative capacity than is found in many less-affluent states. Their findings are based on extensive interviews with the street-level bureaucrats—a research approach that generates powerful insights into how policies actually work on the ground.

The authors find a mix of macro and micro factors that cause what they call an illusion of services—the simultaneous availability of open treatment beds together with obstacles that prevent people from obtaining services when they show up and ask for them. These factors include admission criteria and the framing of opioids under a medical model of care, which causes hospitals to turn away patients who are not displaying outward signs of physical drug withdrawal. Larger, macro policy failures drive these micro issues of scarcity, including federal workforce policies, the lack of physicians eligible to prescribe buprenorphine, and—even more prosaically—staff shortages that led community facilities to turn away people in need, brought about by inadequate pay for people working in underserved areas. In short, the authors identify what the public management literature has long recognized to be bureaucratic goal displacement. Here we return to the disconnect between what policy makers believe is the problem is and how to address it, relative to the problems in actuality. Better use of the tools of policy analysis (define the problem, tailor the solution appropriately, confront the trade-offs) is critical to making tangible and sustainable progress on the opioid and substance abuse problem, yet the role of policy analysis is often neglected in a political process that places a premium on immediate action and symbolic solutions.

The Mediating Role of Partisanship and Information in the Opioid Epidemic

If ever there was a problem begging for officeholders to put partisan needs aside and focus on the public interest, it is the opioid epidemic. The test should be what solutions work—not on which party formulated them. However, the opioid epidemic has unfolded in the United States during an era of rising political polarization in which the two parties have battled over many health policy issues, most notably the enactment of the Affordable Care Act. Competition for power encourages Democrats and Republicans to differentiate themselves from their partisan opponents, even on issues where liberals and conservatives essentially agree (Lee 2009). How much difference has partisanship made in shaping responses to the crisis? To shed light on this important question, Colleen M. Grogan, Clifford S. Bersamira, Phillip M. Singer, Bikki Tran Smith, Harold A. Pollack, Christina M. Andrews, and Amanda J. Abraham investigate whether Democrat-led and Republican-led states have had different or similar responses to the opioid epidemic. Based on a legislative analysis across all 50 states, an online survey of state Medicaid agencies, and in-depth case studies with policy stakeholders, they find that Democratic and Republican states alike have passed legislation to address the opioid crisis, but that the level of fiscal commitment to address the opioid epidemic has been much higher in (predominantly) Democrat-led states that expanded their Medicaid program under the ACA. In Republican-led states that have declined to expand Medicaid, many people suffering from opioid use disorder (OUD) have found themselves without access to treatment.

The opioid crisis does not respect partisan boundaries, of course, and many of the individuals suffering from OUD are part of the GOP's party base. This raises a genuine puzzle. How have Republican officeholders in non-Medicaid-expansion states managed to pursue a policy that denies access to treatment without suffering electorally? Overall, the authors find that state-level Republicans have strategically distanced themselves from Republicans at the federal level. They have also pursued conservative policy options in their existing Medicaid programs, including copays and work requirements, tightened access over opioid prescribing, and adopted targeted expansions for "deserving" populations such as pregnant women. Taken together, these findings help explain how Republican officeholders have managed to claim credit for addressing the opioid crisis without endorsing major new investments in public health spending.

A key intervening variable in this partisan outcome was likely the role of information, a topic to which the study of Paul F. Testa, Susan L. Moffitt, and Marie Schenk contributes key insights. One of the challenges in understanding the influence of information is that people vary in their information exposure and the degree to which they actively seek out information. To capture these complexities, the authors performed an experiment in which some subjects were randomized to receive informational facts about the opioid epidemic and others were given the option of whether to receive the information. The study included three main outcome measures: respondents' objective knowledge about the opioid crisis, beliefs about the primary cause of this crisis, and support for general policy measures to address this issue.

The authors' findings are quite intriguing. They found that people who were interested in receiving more information about the crisis were more likely to have higher levels of education and income, less likely to be racial minorities, and more likely to identify as Democrats and liberals. Those people who would opt to receive information have different views regarding who or what is to blame for the opioid epidemic, with those more interested in finding out about the epidemic more likely to attribute blame to health care providers and less likely to attribute blame to illicit drug use. Finally, the authors show that among people likely to receive this information, information about the crisis "has a large positive effect on increasing support for treatment-oriented policies to address the opioid epidemic but no effect on support for more punitive approaches," whereas the policy preferences of those who would not seek out the information were unchanged. Overall, the study results suggest that the effects of information about the opioid crisis will vary a great deal across the US population, based on the likelihood that a given person will encounter it. A better understanding of these issues could help policy makers design more effective information campaigns that would be better tailored to particular audiences or subgroups.

Conclusion

An overarching question of this special issue is whether and to what extent politics and policy bear a measure of responsibility for the opioid epidemic's severity and duration. Rather than come together against a common threat, policy makers often retreated to their partisan and ideological corners, allowing the epidemic to diffuse across larger and larger segments of the US population. Not only were the perceptions of the causes and solutions to the crisis deeply divided along political lines, the policy investments and administrative capacity building seemed to default on average to a policy response that was too late and too limited. In the global health arena, policy makers and researchers are moving to a more sophisticated and multifaceted understanding of the factors that contribute to effective health systems. They are increasingly recognizing the important role of health system governance. In US health policy, leaders and researchers seem less likely to use political and legal analysis to explain mortality and morbidity outcomes. The essays in this special issue clearly point to the need for public health practitioners and scholars to put political institutions and politics front and center.

Acknowledgment

Miriam Laugesen acknowledges the support of the Tow Foundation.

References

Berger, Peter L., and Thomas Luckman. 1966. *The Social Construction of Knowledge*. New York: Doubleday.

Case, Anne, and Angus Deaton. 2015. "Rising Morbidity and Mortality in Midlife among White Non-Hispanic Americans in the 21st Century." *Proceedings of the National Academy of Sciences* 112, no. 49: 15078–83.

DiAngelo, Robin. 2012. "Chapter 10: What Makes Racism So Hard for Whites to See?" *Counterpoints* 398: 167–89.

Gilens, Martin. 1999. *Why Americans Hate Welfare: Race, Media, and the Politics of Antipoverty Policy*. Chicago: University of Chicago Press.

Goode, Erich, and Nachman Ben-Yehuda. 1994. "Moral Panics: Culture, Politics, and Social Construction." *Annual Review of Sociology* 20, no. 1: 149–71.

Lee, Frances E. 2009. *Beyond Ideology: Politics, Principles, and Partisanship in the US Senate*. Chicago: University of Chicago Press.

Schneider, Anne, and Ingram, Heken. 1993. "Social Construction of Target Populations: Implications for Politics and Policy." *American Political Science Review* 87, no. 2: 334–47. doi.org/10.2307/2939044

Stone, Deborah A. 2011. *Policy Paradox: The Art of Political Decision Making*. 3rd ed. New York: W. W. Norton and Company.

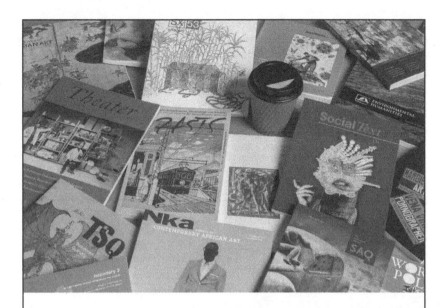

Keep up to date on new scholarship

Issue alerts are a great way to stay current on all the cutting-edge scholarship from your favorite Duke University Press journals. This free service delivers tables of contents directly to your inbox, informing you of the latest groundbreaking work as soon as it is published.

To sign up for issue alerts:

1. Visit **dukeu.press/register** and register for an account. You do not need to provide a customer number.

2. After registering, visit **dukeu.press/alerts**.

3. Go to "Latest Issue Alerts" and click on "Add Alerts."

4. Select as many publications as you would like from the pop-up window and click "Add Alerts."

read.dukeupress.edu/journals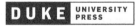

East Asian Science, Technology and Society: An International Journal

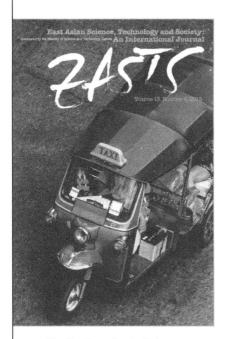

Sponsored by the Ministry of Science and Technology of Taiwan, *EASTS* publishes research on how society and culture in East Asia interact with science, technology, and medicine.

Recent topics include research misconduct, citizen science, network and human, and subimperial formations in East Asia.

For information about submitting to the journal, visit dukeupress.edu/easts *or email* eastsjournal@gmail.com.

Wen-Hua Kuo, *editor in chief*
Sulfikar Amir, Hee-Je Bak, Fa-ti Fan, Yuko Fujigaki, Chihyung Jeon, Sean Hsiang-Lin Lei, Akihisa Setoguchi, Margaret Sleeboom-Faulkner, and Wen-Ling Tu, *associate editors*

Subscribe today.
Quarterly

Individuals $50
Students $25
Single issues $14

dukeupress.edu/easts

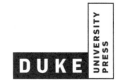